Mothering with Breastfeeding and Maternal Care

Mizin Park Kawasaki, M.D.

iUniverse, Inc.
New York Lincoln Shanghai

Mothering with Breastfeeding and Maternal Care

iUniverse books may be ordered through booksellers or by contacting:

iUniverse
2021 Pine Lake Road, Suite 100
Lincoln, NE 68512
www.iuniverse.com
1-800-Authors (1-800-288-4677)

ISBN-13: 978-0-595-33546-6 (pbk)
ISBN-13: 978-0-595-66965-3 (cloth)
ISBN-13: 978-0-595-78347-2 (ebk)
ISBN-10: 0-595-33546-2 (pbk)
ISBN-10: 0-595-66965-4 (cloth)
ISBN-10: 0-595-78347-3 (ebk)

Printed in the United States of America

For Arnold
and our two children, Lee and Megan,
with love

Contents

ACKNOWLEDGEMENTS

I offer my deepest respect and gratitude to Daisaku and Kaneko Ikeda for their mentorship. Their keen wisdom, intellect, humanity, and compassion encourage and inspire me daily.

The late Ashley Montagu was a wise and brilliant man whose enlightened and articulate view of humanity should be cherished by a much larger audience.

I have only profound gratitude for my beautiful mother, San K. J. Lee, whose indefatigable support and love have helped me to stay home with my children. I offer appreciation to my stepfather, Jules Brassner, for his affection and consistently warm support of my writing.

I appreciate those who perused the vast expanse of the World Wide Web, found my Web site, www.humaneparenting.com, and left thoughtful feedback.

I could not have written this book without the support and encouragement of my husband, Arnold. His unconditional love enriches everyone around him.

Our children, Lee and Megan, are two special human beings who remind me daily why life is meaningful. They have brightened my life immeasurably.

INTRODUCTION

This book is not a guide to parenting, but I hope to provide enough information to encourage parents to consider offering their babies the benefits of both breastfeeding and maternal care. Using a diverse array of references and personal anecdotes, I will argue that babies and young children need and deserve the intimacy of breastfeeding and maternal care.

In recent years it has become politically incorrect to acknowledge the singular importance of a woman's presence in her child's life. Some feminists even denounce mother-infant bonding and assert that maternal care is no different from safe and somewhat educational care offered by anyone else. The widespread disregard for both breastfeeding and maternal care during early childhood may arguably be unprecedented in human history.

This book is a defense of the unique role women play in young children's lives. It is divided into two parts: the first half advocates breastfeeding, and the second half defends stay-at-home mothering. The two subjects may appear to be unrelated, but they are integrally connected. Throughout the long history of human existence, the majority of women nearly always breastfed and remained close to their babies. It has been only within the past century that the art of breastfeeding was nearly eliminated from the American way of life. Concurrently, it has become acceptable over the past two decades for the majority of women to deny their babies and young children the benefits of maternal care.

Readers should note that I am not offering a definitive analysis of breastfeeding, stay-at-home mothering, or family life. There are numerous textbooks and informative books that elucidate in detail the vast benefits of breastfeeding; books and local and nationwide organizations that support stay-at-home mothering; and many scholarly books that analyze family life. What I am attempting to do is to clarify how profoundly important both breastfeeding and maternal care are to the well-being of children, women, men, and family life as a whole.

This book will not suit everyone, but I would have enjoyed reading this kind of book, especially when my children were younger. As a woman who chose to stay home full-time with two children, I found that most extant books on child-rearing were either diametrically opposed to or not nearly supportive enough of my thoughts on parenting. On a positive note I did find a most inspiring book in

1995 when I came across *The Natural Superiority of Women* by Ashley Montagu, the well-known scientist and anthropologist.

Ashley Montagu's book was inspirational, and I wrote him a letter of gratitude. Despite his advanced age and busy schedule, he was kind enough to reply. We corresponded over the next four years, during which time he was gracious enough to mail me copies of his articles and books. He also sent me books by other authors, including one by the late historian and social critic Christopher Lasch. Ashley Montagu passed away at the age of 94 in late 1999.

Over the past several years, I have read many books by Ashley Montagu and Christopher Lasch. Their work is of incomparable significance, and their ideas should be shared continually with others. Both of these highly intellectual and astute men had a profound understanding of women and the unique contributions women have made and continue to make to humanity. I hope to offer a meaningful discussion of some of the brilliant thoughts and analyses both men brought to light on the subjects of children, women, family life, and work life. The contents of this book, however, reflect my personal opinions and not necessarily those of either Ashley Montagu or Christopher Lasch.

Fundamentally, I contend that modern child-rearing practices should include breastfeeding and maternal care. Women need to play an active and indispensable role in child-rearing, especially during early childhood. I realize that this suggestion conflicts with popular assumptions of what women are supposed to accomplish in life. Additionally, there are countless situations in which women are obligated to work outside the home. My mother, for example, worked both inside and outside the home in order to earn an income throughout my childhood. Obviously, not all women will be able to stay home with their children, but parents should consider thoughtfully and deliberately a woman's irreplaceable role in her young child's life.

Some readers may perceive my advocacy of breastfeeding and stay-at-home mothering to be a response to my personal experiences as a latchkey kid. This is, however, a superficial understanding of my views and reasoning. I have accumulated knowledge and wisdom over the years from various sources, including my educational and professional training, reading widely, interacting with other parents, and breastfeeding and staying home with my children. It is my ardent wish to share with others what I have learned because I think that a woman's role in child-rearing is woefully underestimated and underappreciated in modern society. It is a shame that mothering has become so misunderstood over the past century.

Christopher Lasch observed that the failure to appreciate mothering as a worthy contribution to the well-being of family life and society at large did not occur incidentally. At the turn of the twentieth century, various professionals (including educators, social workers, psychiatrists, physicians, psychologists, and penologists) claimed to know more about child-rearing than the women who bore the children. Concerted efforts were made to strip women of motherly intuition, knowledge, and wisdom related to child-rearing. The imputation was that parents were no longer capable of rearing their children without the guidance of child-rearing experts.

After a century of such misguided ideology, many parents today feel inept and unable to care for their own babies and children; they feel compelled to seek advice from more knowledgeable sources. This does not mean, however, that such sources offer more wisdom and compassion for either babies or their parents. Even so, parental dependency upon external child-rearing guidance has replaced parental self-sufficiency. Such a significant change in child-rearing practices did not occur by chance, of course, since this was an important goal not only of child-rearing professionals but also of pioneering feminists who no longer wished to remain bound to home and family.

I will clarify that I am not offering an indictment of feminism since I have gained an education and profession because of the women's movement. I am, however, echoing Christopher Lasch's challenge to feminists. Simply stated, feminists should do more to help women fulfill their responsibilities as mothers and homemakers. This is especially imperative since the modern feminist vision of women seems to preclude breastfeeding and maternal care. I hope to offer enough evidence and thoughtful criticism to encourage parents to think differently and more positively about the significance of their participation in early child care.

I hope that my defense of breastfeeding and maternal care inspires individuals to seek to parent in a way that truly considers the well-being of infants and children first. Babies and children need to be reared with the loving maternal care that should be their birthright. Unfortunately, contemporary mothering neglects the importance of mother-infant bonding. It is time to take a somber look at why standards of mothering are so low and elevate them so that more young babies and children can receive the benefits of breastfeeding and maternal care.

PART I

LEARNING THE ART OF BREASTFEEDING

1

BECOMING A MOTHER

A MOTHER BY CHOICE

In 1988, I was newly wed and in my last year of pediatric residency. I looked forward to becoming a mother, and I was sure that I could become pregnant, have a baby, and return to work fairly immediately. The timing seemed to be right since I could have the baby the summer before I would begin working full-time as a practicing pediatrician.

Over the long course of medical school and pediatric residency, I observed many women physicians who became pregnant, had babies, and returned to work outside the home. For example, during medical school, I once saw a pregnant surgical resident lay on a gurney to rest for a few moments after she endured a grueling day of work and night call. Even though this resident experienced complications with her pregnancy, she managed to take off only a week from work before giving birth. She then quickly resumed her normal call schedule, completed her residency, and started a specialty fellowship in Plastic Surgery. Like nearly all the other women physicians I knew, motherhood and a young baby at home did not stop this woman from returning to work outside the home.

I assumed that I would follow in the footsteps of these women physicians, and this is still what I thought when I finally did become pregnant. By then I was working with two other pediatricians in private practice. The owner of the practice saw no difficulty in accommodating a lighter work schedule for me. He even suggested kindly and thoughtfully that I put a crib in the office, so I could bring the baby with me to work. I had heard about a pediatrician in New York whose six children had roamed freely in her office while she practiced medicine; I thought that I could perhaps work out a similar arrangement.

Nine years after I left the practice to stay home full-time, I ran into a nurse and a bookkeeper who still worked at the pediatric office I had left. Apparently, they had suspected early on that I probably did not have the drive or interest to become a supermom. Thus, they were not at all surprised that I chose to stay home with my baby.

It is remarkable how differently people will perceive a given individual's capabilities. One of my closest friends was utterly confident that I would and should become a supermom. She had a friend who worked full-time as a dentist, had two or three children at home, and managed to maintain her home well and efficiently. Her friend always prepared and froze a week's worth of meals on the weekends, so her family could eat home-cooked meals during the week. After hearing about the virtues of this accomplished woman, I agreed that I could surely do the same.

I disappointed my friend since I did exactly the opposite of what she expected. I stopped working as a pediatrician after my first child's preterm birth. I simply could not return to work immediately. As I took my scheduled four-month maternity leave, I expected to adapt to the change of having a baby and returning to work outside the home. The adjustment did not occur, and I wound up staying home indefinitely.

Over the fourteen years I have stayed home, an assortment of friends, family, and strangers have wondered about my decision to stop working outside the home. For example, when my son was about four months old, one of my husband's co-workers asked when I would resume my medical practice. He was astonished that I had given up my work to stay home with a baby. He thought that anybody could stay home, including his wife, but he could not fathom why an educated physician would do so. He predicted that if I chose to stay home, then I would probably have many children. When he learned several years later that I had only two children, he simply shook his head in confusion. I have confounded many people with my decision to stay home.

UNPREPARED FOR PRETERM LABOR

I was 29 years old, in good health, and seven months pregnant when I went into labor suddenly and unexpectedly. My husband and I were watching television on a Sunday night when I began to feel pain. As much as I had hoped that I was experiencing a bout of upset stomach, a bit of spotting alarmed me. We called my obstetrician and followed her advice to go to the hospital.

Once we arrived at the hospital, I received the kind of conventional medical care I dispensed regularly to others throughout my medical training. I was a pediatrician who was steeped in the culture of hospital birthing, and I trusted the system in which I was trained. I also viewed my pregnancy and childbirth as medical conditions, so it did not even occur to me to seek the care of anyone other than a Board certified obstetrician.

Long after I had my children, I learned about women who birthed their babies alone and others who used midwives. I was astounded to learn that a friend of mine had reached down during labor and helped her newborn emerge from the birth canal. My friend understood clearly how powerful she was as a woman giving birth, and she demonstrated her ability to take charge of her child's birth.

In contrast, I was simply uneducated about natural childbirth. I understood childbirth from the perspective of hospital birthing, so this meant that I experienced the opposite of empowerment during my son's birth: I participated passively during childbirth and did as I was told.

HOSPITAL BIRTHING

Historically, women gave birth at home without anesthesia and in the presence of a midwife and family members. According to historians Dorothy and Carl J. Schneider (1994, 157–159), a small minority of early twentieth century American women thought they would be gaining greater control over their bodies by advocating changes in prevalent childbirth practices. They managed to generate an enormous amount of attention from the press by gathering at diverse places, including public rallies and department stores, to inform women about the use of anesthesia during childbirth.

Wealthy women like Mrs. John Jacob Astor traveled to Germany to give birth under an anesthesia regimen called the "twilight sleep." They received morphine at the beginning of labor and then a dose of memory-destroying scopolamine, followed by ether or chloroform when the fetus was in the birth canal (1994, 158). The women would writhe in pain during the birth but would have no memory of the event. If they suffered no complications, they would awaken from sleep and receive their babies without recalling the labor and birth.

Women lobbied for hospital birthing as opposed to home birthing, the care of doctors instead of midwives, and anesthetic relief for the pain of labor. The lobbying efforts of this small minority of women were highly successful, but women did not necessarily gain greater control over their bodies. The institution of mandatory hospital birthing and the eradication of home birthing were actually costly to women. No longer were women surrounded by loving family members in the comfort of their homes while giving birth.

Healthy pregnant women were to give birth to healthy babies in the confines of hospitals that were filled with sick patients. Instead of being reassured by experienced midwives who did not use anesthesia, pregnant women were now in the hands of physicians who were often inexpert in baby birthing and sometimes too eager to speed the birth process with the use of forceps and cesarean intervention.

THE PREVALENCE OF CESAREAN SECTIONS

Since hospital birthing is now standard practice, the majority of women participate in childbirth passively. A growing minority of women are even promoting hospital practices that violate the integrity of the birthing process. For example, I once had a neighbor who went to great lengths to assure that only her long-time physician would deliver her second baby.

My neighbor's physician was scheduled to go on vacation around her due date, so he suggested that she be induced to give birth a week earlier. She complied, but the hospitalization and induction failed since the baby was not ready to be born. Her physician returned from his vacation and eventually delivered the baby, who was now overdue, via cesarean section. As my neighbor relayed the details of her baby's birth, she spoke as if every woman experiences this type of childbirth.

The reality is that too many women experience childbirth as my neighbor did. Many years ago when I was on call for my pediatric group, I noticed that one obstetrician had three cesarean sections scheduled for a Friday evening. A nurse informed me that the cesarean sections, including a preterm delivery, were scheduled because the obstetrician was leaving for an overseas trip the following morning. Although none of these women had to give birth that night, they trusted their doctor enough to give birth via cesarean section.

A cesarean section is major abdominal surgery wherein an incision is made through the abdominal skin, connective tissue, muscles, and the uterus in order to extract a newborn. It is a procedure that cuts through healthy skin and tissues; invades the normally sterile abdominal cavity; and creates an artificial opening for the uterus, an organ that is not meant to be incised since the cervix provides a natural exit for the emerging fetus. Every woman should examine intraoperative pictures of a cesarean section before she chooses to undergo the procedure electively.

My husband has a friend who decided twice to give birth via elective cesarean section because she was nearing the age of forty, and she thought she was too old to give birth vaginally. A brief examination of Farook Al-Azzawi's *Color Atlas of Childbirth and Obstetric Techniques*, which includes graphic photographs and descriptions of how an obstetrician performs a cesarean section, might have convinced her to choose otherwise. At certain points in the book, the author recommends tearing tissue with fingers instead of incising it with a scalpel.

The incision for the cesarean section must necessarily be large since a baby needs to be removed through the surgical opening. Since most general surgical procedures can now be carried out through small incisions, it is egregious that a surgical procedure that is performed only on women and that is as invasive as the cesarean section continues to be done routinely. While few patients would risk major abdominal surgery unless a serious illness requires the removal of a diseased or cancerous internal organ, many healthy pregnant women choose to undergo elective cesarean sections.

In an effort to decrease the risks associated with cesarean deliveries, a national U.S. health objective for the year 2000 was to reduce the overall rate of cesarean delivery to less than or equal to 15 percent (Centers for Disease Control 1995). The risks of a cesarean section to the mother include infection at the site of the incision, the urinary tract, or the uterine lining; hemorrhage at the site of incision or placental attachment to the uterus; anemia and possible need for a blood transfusion; possible injury to other organs, such as the bladder or bowel; blood clots; complications from anesthesia; psychological difficulties; and maternal mortality four times greater than that for a vaginal birth. The risks of a cesarean section to the baby include possible preterm birth because of inaccurate dates; respiratory distress syndrome, which is associated with high morbidity; delayed bonding with mother; and delayed introduction to breastfeeding. Despite these risks, the cesarean section is the most commonly performed surgical procedure in U.S. hospitals, and efforts to curtail its use have been unsuccessful.

According to an August 2, 2005, Reuters article entitled "C-section most common hospital procedure-study," 1.2 million cesarean operations were performed in 2003 at a cost of $14.6 billion in the U.S. More cesarean sections were performed in U.S. hospitals than any other surgical procedure. The preliminary data for the year 2003 showed that 27.6 percent of all U.S. births were delivered by cesarean section (Centers for Disease Control 2004a). In contrast, the rate was 4.5 percent in 1965 (Cesarean Childbirth 2005).

Over a quarter of babies are now born via cesarean section even though there is an increased risk of maternal death and morbidity, as well as perinatal morbidity. The increased rate of cesarean section births reflects many obstetricians' hesitation to permit women to give birth vaginally after they have had an earlier cesarean section. This is the case even though numerous studies demonstrate the safety of such births. The rate of cesarean sections is also increased by the strong demand for epidural pain relief during childbirth.

A May 2005 study in *Obstetrics and Gynecology* found an increased rate of cesarean section among women who received epidural analgesia (Lieberman et al. 2005). Of 1,562 pregnant women examined, a high percentage (92 percent) received epidural analgesia. The authors of the study concluded the following: the fetus changed its position during labor; the administration of epidural analgesia increased by four-fold the probability that the fetus would turn its head and emerge face-up instead of face-down; and there was a ten-fold increase in the likelihood of a cesarean section if the fetus was positioned face-up as compared to face-down. The reality may be that an overwhelming percentage of women in labor request epidural pain relief, but few women comprehend how significantly such pain relief increases their risk of undergoing cesarean section.

The cesarean section clearly should be reserved for true emergencies when the life of either the mother or the fetus is endangered. As it stands, though, it hardly seems possible that emergencies occur so frequently that more than one-quarter of U.S. births require cesarean surgical intervention. The need for a cesarean section should be considered with caution, especially by those women who have the option of refusing one.

THE SIGNIFICANCE OF LABOR DURING CHILDBIRTH

Some women may choose an elective cesarean section because they fear the pain of labor and prefer to avoid it even at the cost of undergoing major abdominal surgery. Increasingly, the labor of childbirth is assessed to be unnecessary because its sole objective appears to be the emergence of the viable newborn. Hence, some women think that they can avoid the pain and suffering of labor by extracting the newborn via elective cesarean section. This view of labor, however, fails to appreciate the utterly indispensable role labor plays in preparing the fetus for the transition from life in the womb to life outside the womb.

The anthropologist Ashley Montagu discusses in depth the significance of labor during childbirth in his book *Touching: The Human Significance of the Skin*. He offers the following important insight (1986, 57): "Birth represents a complex and highly important series of functional changes which serve to prepare the newborn for the passage across the bridge between gestation within the womb and gestation outside the womb." Ashley Montagu clarifies that labor is essential in helping to prepare the baby's body to begin functioning completely on its own after birth.

The powerful and painful uterine contractions that constitute labor act to massage the skin of the fetus. It is the critical stimulation of fetal skin during labor that activates the baby's life-sustaining systems. These systems are the nervous, respiratory, cardiovascular, gastrointestinal, genitourinary, immunological, and endocrine systems. Without the proper stimulation of these vital systems, it becomes that much more difficult for a newborn to make a smooth transition to life outside the womb. Ashley Montagu comments that the labor of human beings is longer than the labor of other mammals primarily to ensure the adequate tactile stimulation of the fetus prior to birth.

The skin is an important organ, and it is also the largest organ in the human body. The skin arises from the ectoderm, which is the same embryonic tissue from which the entire nervous system arises. The skin and the nervous system are, therefore, intimately connected. Located throughout the skin are sensory nerves which receive stimuli from the environment and send impulses to the brain and spinal cord. In turn, messages are relayed from the brain and spinal cord at the proper levels via the autonomic nervous system to the organs which participate in the life-sustaining systems. The uterine contractions during labor stimulate the skin of the fetus and the nerves that activate the baby's essential life-sustaining systems.

Non-human mammals provide their newborns with sufficient tactile stimulation by licking them soon after birth (Montagu 1986, 23). For example, it has been noted that a newborn kitten must receive tactile stimulation in the area between the genitalia and the anus. Without such stimulation, the kitten will probably die as a result of a failure of either the genitourinary or the gastrointestinal system. Instinctive licking on the part of animal mothers apparently helps to ensure activation of the vital organ systems of their newborns.

In contrast, human beings do not possess the genetic determination to lick their newborns. In the absence of such an instinct, the labor of childbirth serves as the primary source of adequate tactile stimulation for the human fetus (Montagu 1986, 29). Comprehending the significance of labor from this perspective may enable more women to endure better the hardship and pain associated with giving birth.

THE EPISIOTOMY: AN INVASIVE PROCEDURE

My preterm labor progressed despite my obstetrician's attempts to stop it with medical intervention. She considered seriously the idea of performing a cesarean section, but a perinatologist who specialized in high-risk obstetrics deliveries convinced her that it was unnecessary. My obstetrician then proceeded to incise a huge episiotomy in order to allow my preterm baby's small head to pass easily through the birth canal. The episiotomy was so large that even the assisting nurse was surprised enough to mention her concern aloud.

An episiotomy is a cut in the perineum, which is the tissue between the vaginal opening and the anus. An anesthetic is injected directly into the tissue before it is cut, and there is some bleeding. The incision is usually made with a pair of scissors and is intended to "prevent the posterior vulval tissue from suffering excessive distension by the fetal head" and replace "a ragged vaginal and perineal tear with neat, clean-cut tissue, which facilitates optimal repair" (Al-Azzawi 1990, 37). The episiotomy is supposed to prevent excessive stretching of muscles and tissues as the baby's head descends into the birth canal, and it also provides a straight incision that is easier to sew closed.

In *Natural Childbirth the Bradley Way*, Susan McCutcheon (1996, 189–192) discusses her concerns about episiotomies. As an experienced childbirth educator, she notes that most women do not need episiotomies. During labor the perineum is stretched to the point where a natural anesthesia occurs due to numbing of the nerves in that area prior to crowning. In this naturally anesthetized state and as labor progresses, the thinned perineal tissue may remain intact, or spontaneous tears may occur painlessly. McCutcheon writes that many spontaneous tears heal far more rapidly than do incisions made with scissors. She points out that episiotomies, which may involve a fairly thick layer of tissue, may even lead to sexual dysfunction if the wound heals poorly. Episiotomies, from her perspective, are far from benign.

The *Journal of the American Medical Association* recently published a review of 26 episiotomy studies done over the course of more than five decades. The conclusion of the review was the following: "Evidence does not support maternal benefits traditionally ascribed to routine episiotomy" (Hartmann et al. 2005). Episiotomy was not found to decrease women's risk of injury, healing time, or experience of pain. Women also did not experience less pain with intercourse. The review found that spontaneous tears are smaller and have no need for sutures. According to an *Associated Press* article by Carla K. Johnson on May 4, 2005, the review's lead author, Dr. Katherine Hartmann, estimates that one million women undergo the unnecessary procedure each year.

I would have endured anything for my son at the time of his birth, and I raised no objections to the episiotomy. I viewed it as being an inevitable part of childbirth because I had seen episiotomies performed so often before. If I had educated myself a bit better, I might have responded differently to our situation.

When things go awry during pregnancy and childbirth, however, parents generally accept their doctors' recommendations without reservation. The priority is, after all, to ensure the safety and well-being of the newborn. Hence, I trusted my doctor and hoped for the best outcome as my labor continued.

DEHUMANIZING HOSPITAL CARE

Even though I felt the pain of the labor throughout the birthing experience, I had been distracted by the medical interventions. When I was finally given permission to push my baby out, I began to feel the true impact of labor. The powerful contractions were sending the baby further down the birth canal, and they were excruciatingly painful. Facing the pain head-on was a great challenge and, although the pushing did not last long, I was prepared to close up shop near the end and leave without giving birth.

Only years later did I comprehend how significant those contractions were for the well-being of our baby. He did as well as he did during his hospitalization because he received a significant amount of tactile stimulation during labor. He was that much more prepared to face the difficult transition from life in the womb to life outside the womb.

I was permitted to hold my son only briefly before he was whisked off to the Neonatal Intensive Care Unit (NICU). He breathed well initially, but the neonatologist found that his breathing had become labored in the NICU. She intubated him; attached him to a ventilator; placed intravenous lines into his arms, navel, and feet; inserted a painful urinary catheter to measure his urine output; and hooked him up to cardiac and respiratory monitors. When I finally saw my son again, he was attached to tubes, wires, and machines.

All of this was evidently for his good, but it was difficult to see him in this condition. His small limbs and body parts had already been poked frequently with needles and catheters, his delicate skin was covered with adhesive pads and tape that connected him to monitors and IV sites, and the endotracheal tube that was taped to his face went through his mouth and into his trachea to force oxygenated air into his lungs. Although I had been able to dispense similar care with relative equanimity as a physician, it was a different experience to see my small son receive such care.

To make matters worse, the young nurse taking care of my son seemed indifferent to my baby's ordeal. I was perturbed profoundly by the way she handled him. At one point, she casually lifted his foot and dropped it while she recounted what had been done to him. Astounded by her disrespect for my son, I muttered that she should treat him more gently. My comment, however, made it less likely that she would handle him with greater care.

The following morning, another nurse greeted me less than cordially by saying, "Wipe that sad look off your face." The casual and cruel nature of the remark caught me off guard. It was true that my son was doing well, but I was still saddened immeasurably by my inability to help him. Additionally, I was hardly reassured by the nurses who were treating him not as a small human being but almost like a specimen. It was all so dehumanizing, and I could do nothing for him.

BEREFT WITHOUT MY SON

After my son's release from the hospital, the neonatologist who cared for him for six weeks dictated a discharge summary for "Baby Girl Kawasaki." Apparently, my son was simply another patient of indeterminate sex who experienced typical neonatal problems. How could I explain to everyone, however, that my son was not just another neonate?

During the many months of my pregnancy, my son had been an intimate part of my life. In fact, he should still have been inside my womb instead of outside the womb without me. He would have been safe inside the womb; instead, he was in the hands of a staff trained to do procedures. Although the majority of nurses and respiratory therapists were sympathetic and kind, it is still difficult to forget the disturbing insensitivity of the nurses I encountered during the first twenty-four hours of my son's life.

His hospitalization was prolonged, and it was depressing and discouraging to be separated from my son for so long. Even though I was optimistic about my son's health and his eventual release from the hospital, we had no idea how long he would be hospitalized. Forty days seemed interminable. As we waited for his improvement and eventual discharge from the hospital, the long days revolved around visiting him in the hospital and pumping my breasts. Even though I felt intuitively that our separation was far from healthy, I was unable to articulate the complexity of my emotions.

I felt both sad and helpless. My sister recalled how I draped my entire body over my son's plastic isolette during one visit. It was an odd but telling gesture: I wanted to shield him, but I couldn't. My son's preterm birth was intimidating: I felt distanced from him even though I would sit next to him and hold his little hand or foot for hours. In truth, I was afraid to touch him for fear of transmitting germs to him or disturbing him.

Fortunately, current approaches to caring for preterm babies include encouraging early and intimate contact between preterm baby and parent. The practice of Kangaroo Care entails placing infants atop their mothers' chests to receive skin-to-skin contact for prolonged periods as soon as possible after birth. These infants have been shown to "maintain stable skin temperatures, respiratory rates, and oxygen saturation levels" (Harrison 2001). Gentle and still touch that is unrelated to procedures performed by medical personnel reduces preterm infants' stress and increases their level of comfort.

Although my son and I were a dyad, we were neither physically nor emotionally attuned to one another. This was both sad and ironic since it was the wonder of the mother-newborn dyad that drew me to pediatrics in medical school. Every morning during my obstetrics clinical rotation, the residents and medical students visited the women who had recently given birth. Invariably, I was impressed and uplifted by the sight of universally radiant and beautiful mothers cradling cherubic newborns in their arms. For thousands of years, poets and artists have been moved to depict the beauty and intimacy of the mother-infant dyad. Disappointingly, I did not feel at all radiant, and I could not even hold my son in my arms for the first several days of his life.

I felt bereft without my son. The birth had been profoundly impersonal since it took place in a room filled with hospital personnel who anticipated a disastrous birth. Fortunately, it became evident soon after the birth that my son and I would be relatively fine. The nurses became preoccupied with other pregnant women in labor, and my husband escorted my mother and stepfather back to their hotel. In the middle of the night, as I lay alone in my hospital bed, my life felt incredibly empty. My son had come out of the womb far too early, and it felt so wrong to be without him.

FORCED SEPARATION

Most babies in the United States are born in hospitals that have established the protocol of forced separation. The separation of newborns from their mothers immediately after birth is fairly standard practice since the needs of mothers and their newborns are considered separately. There are even two sets of nurses: maternity nurses care for the mothers while pediatric nurses care for the newborns. The separation of care may be so complete in some hospitals that the maternity ward and the nursery may be at opposite ends of long corridors or on different floors.

Healthy newborn babies are taken away from their mothers so that hospital personnel may complete paperwork. Of course, it is important to identify newborns correctly since unintentional mistakes and deliberate misdeeds may result in switched babies. It is fairly simple and practical, however, to examine a healthy baby in his mother's arms even if it may be a bit inconvenient for the nurses and doctors. One would think that paperwork should be secondary to the well-being of both mothers and newborns.

Regrettably, few hospital personnel think twice before separating the newborn from his mother in the delivery room. A doctor, nurse, or respiratory therapist often evaluates the newborn prior to allowing his mother to hold her baby. Newborns delivered via cesarean sections are shown briefly to their mothers before they are carted off to be examined, dried, and measured in a different section of the hospital. The nurses and doctors explain matter-of-factly that it is for the good of the baby and the mother that they are separated. Frequently, a mother is left to think alone about her baby as the baby's father scurries off to escort the newborn elsewhere and far away from his mother.

The separation of mother from newborn occurs in the majority of births in the U.S. Although it is a mother's right to remain close to her newborn, she may be criticized for wanting to be with her baby. Thus, a mother who does not wish to be separated from her newborn may be labeled by nursing staff as being "uncooperative," "pushy," or "demanding." In the artificial realm of hospital culture, it may be impractical for a mother to be intimately bound to her newborn.

This is unfortunate since early mother-infant intimacy helps to establish a healthy mother-infant bond. In the July 23, 1996, issue of the *New York Times*, Natalie Angier explains in her article, "Why Babies Are Born Facing Backward, Helpless and Chubby," that babies appear as they do at birth in order to compel parents to fall in love with them. In the article, anthropologist Sarah Blaffer Hrdy suggests that the human infant acquires layers of fat just before birth for cosmetic reasons.

Although it would be more practical for a thin baby to emerge from the womb, babies are born plumper (and thus, cuter) so that parents will want to care for them. This normal bonding process may be interrupted, however, if a mother is permitted to see her baby for only a few seconds before the baby is wheeled off to a nursery. One may surmise that the separation of the mother-infant dyad in the immediate post-partum period may possibly deny a mother the opportunity to fall in love with her own baby.

2

THE IMMATURE AND NEEDY NEWBORN

BIRTH: A NEWBORN'S TRANSITION

Birth is the singular event that announces the arrival of an independent human being. This view of birth emphasizes the individuality of the newborn and her separation from the mother who gives birth to her. Therefore, as soon as the baby is born, the umbilical cord that connects the newborn to the placenta is clamped and cut, either without ado by the obstetrician or with pride and ceremony by the baby's father.

For the most part, a newborn is welcomed into the world not as an individual who should be kept close to her mother but as a ward of hospital protocol. Hospital protocol entails placing identification bracelets on the newborn's extremities, procuring her footprints, drying her, weighing and measuring her, dressing her with tee shirt and diaper, obtaining blood from her heel to test for hereditary diseases, and placing her into a plastic cart. Amid the excitement of the newborn's arrival, parents are happy to comply with hospital protocol.

In recent years hospitals have modified protocol a bit in response to growing women's demand to make the hospital birthing experience less institutional. Some hospitals now provide a more home-like ambience: the walls of the birthing rooms may be painted in warm colors, and the rooms may be decorated with comfortable furniture. Mothers are also permitted to room-in with their babies by request.

Many newborns, however, are still settled in nurseries. Ashley Montagu comments that the newborn suffers separation from her mother and "is consigned to another room, quaintly called the 'nursery' presumably because no nursing is done in it" (1979, 196). The nursery is often a storage area for newborns since many mothers neither breastfeed their newborns nor feel compelled to be near them. Although today's birthing experiences may be more comfortable for women, most newborns still experience the institutional protocol of being taken away from their mothers immediately after birth.

THE IMMATURE NEWBORN

Birth is actually part of a continuum that begins with conception. For nearly nine months, or 266 1/2 days as Ashley Montagu specifies, a pregnant woman carries her fetus in the womb (1986, 54). The nine months that are normally associated with pregnancy in the womb is the *uterogestation* (Montagu 1961). By all appearances, a nine-month pregnancy must be the right amount of time for the human fetus to develop into an entity mature enough to be born. Why else would a human newborn emerge from the womb after nine months?

In an enlightening discussion of human development, Ashley Montagu explains that the human newborn at birth is very immature (1961). Parents understand this intuitively since they handle their newborn with great care. They are afraid perhaps that insufficient support of the baby's wobbly head and neck might cause damage to his delicate nervous system. They also notice that the newborn is hardly capable of doing much except to suckle, cry, urinate, eliminate, and sleep. The human newborn is completely dependent upon his environment for nourishment, comfort, warmth, touch, cleansing, and protection because he is truly immature.

Compared to other animals, like the newborn elephant and the fallow deer that can run with their herd, the human infant is born in an immature condition (Montagu 1961). These animals have long gestations presumably because they are not predatory, and they need to protect themselves from predators soon after birth. After long gestations, these animals are born in a fairly mature state. Although human beings also have a comparatively long gestation, the human infant finds himself at birth and for long afterward to be wholly dependent upon his caregivers.

As human beings evolved to become upright and bipedal, walking with two legs and two feet, the human brain grew larger while the pelvic outlet became smaller. At birth, the fetus' head must be small enough to pass through the birth canal. If the head is too large, the lives of both mother and newborn will be imperiled. In order to ensure a reasonable head size at birth, then, the newborn's brain must be far from fully grown and developed when he emerges from the womb. Ashley Montagu summarizes the situation succinctly when he describes the human newborn as being "half-done."

It is in this immature state that the newborn needs to experience a transition from dependency in the womb to independence in a vastly different environment. Ashley Montagu (1986, 59) explains that this is a gradual transition: "What the fetus must be prepared to deal with during the birth process is the *immediate* neonatal period of the first few hours, then days, weeks, and months of gradual adjustment and habituation to the requirements of early postnatal existence." Although the newborn may look like a complete individual, he is an immature human being who must adjust to functioning independently of the womb after birth.

IN SUPPORT OF THE MOTHER-INFANT DYAD

A woman makes tremendous sacrifices during pregnancy for the well-being of the fetus in her womb. Not only does her body accommodate the presence of the fetus, but a pregnant woman also experiences alterations in nearly every aspect of her life. Her body shape, bodily functions, appetite, mood, sex drive, social life, physical endurance, and more are all affected by pregnancy. It is not just for anyone that women would undergo so many profound life changes. Most women endure the significant changes that accompany pregnancy and childbirth because the end product is expected to be a healthy newborn.

The many changes wrought by pregnancy, no matter how unaffected many healthy pregnant women appear to be, mark the beginning of a new relationship: the mother-infant dyad. From conception onward, the mother and the life forming in her womb are inseparable since the environment of the womb is created by a living mother, and it sustains the life of the fetus. A healthy woman's womb provides the optimal environment in which her fetus will grow and develop.

In comparison, an unhealthy pregnant woman may present her fetus with an unhealthy womb. For example, the deleterious effects of cigarette smoking during pregnancy were documented long ago. Four decades ago, Ashley Montagu cited numerous studies that describe how cigarette smoking affects adversely the well-being of the fetus. Cigarette smoking reduces the availability of oxygen to the fetus; increases the fetus' exposure to noxious gases such as carbon monoxide; subjects the fetus to the effects of nicotine; and reduces blood flow to the fetus, thereby perhaps reducing the delivery of oxygen and nutrients that are critical to healthy fetal growth and development (Montagu 1965, 100–116).

Dr. R.C. Lowe noted in the 1950s that there had been no significant decrease in the rate of prematurity at a time when prenatal care was improving. He then made the astute observation that the benefits of improved prenatal health care were probably negated by the prevalence of cigarette smoking among pregnant women (Montagu 1965, 107). For instance, the highly admired former First Lady Jacqueline Kennedy Onassis smoked cigarettes surreptitiously throughout a pregnancy that resulted in the sad preterm birth and death of a baby boy.

Several decades ago, most women were given no hope if a baby was born preterm (defined as being born before 37 weeks gestation). I know a woman who retrieved her preterm newborn son from the garbage can after he was discarded by hospital personnel back in the 1960s. They told her that he would never survive, but he grew up to become a healthy and intelligent adult.

With the advent of significant technological advances, it is virtually assured that most newborns will survive outside the womb even if they are born preterm (although their quality of life cannot be guaranteed). A preterm newborn can breathe with the assistance of a respirator; she can also receive a synthetic form of Surfactant, a substance that improves lung function. If the preterm baby cannot tolerate oral feedings, she can be given water, essential proteins, fat, sugar, electrolytes, and minerals through intravenous infusion. If she becomes anemic, she may receive blood transfusions. If she develops bacterial infections, antibiotics can be administered. These are only some of the ways in which preterm newborns can be supported to live outside the womb. In other words, an enormous amount of work must be performed in order to simulate the tasks that are achieved seemingly so effortlessly by a woman's body during a healthy pregnancy.

THE NEWBORN'S NEED FOR AN EXTERNAL WOMB

After nine months of *uterogestation*, childbirth marks the newborn's transition from life within the womb to life outside the womb. The newborn is, in effect, in nearly the same condition as he was before birth except that he is now outside the womb. In his immature state, he is apparently able to function independently of his mother. A newborn, however, is a helpless individual who is utterly dependent upon his environment for survival.

Like the human newborn, the baby kangaroo is also born immature. The joey, however, has the advantage of residing in an external womb whereas the immature human baby does not. The mother kangaroo has a physical pouch that provides her joey with both protection and immediate access to the breasts for nursing. In comparison, the immature human newborn must grow and develop outside the womb in the absence of a maternal pouch.

Ideally, the human infant needs another nine months of gestation outside the womb called a period of *exterogestation* (Montagu 1986, 54). During *exterogestation,* the infant has many needs that must be satisfied, including the need to sleep, be nourished, kept clean and warm, be carried and touched, and be loved and cared for with affection. All these requirements and more for healthy living can be fulfilled only by those who are in the infant's environment.

Throughout most of human history, mothers understood intuitively why they should carry their newborns close to their bodies. In *Untouched: The Need for Genuine Affection in an Impersonal World*, Mariana Caplan describes cultures in which babies are routinely carried on their mothers' backs. Undoubtedly, baby carrying has been an integral part of parenting for most of human history for a sound reason.

A mother's arms and her breasts provide the newborn with a "womb with a view," a term coined with wit by Ashley Montagu. The majority of mothers have always been adept at going about their daily lives while they carried their babies in their arms or on their backs. The modern tendency may be to shun the carrying of babies, but women of yore always carried their babies.

Anthropological studies of indigenous people who live in remote parts of the world as hunter-gatherers reflect a lifestyle that was prevalent prior to civilization as we know it. The following passage describes the !Kung San of Botswana:

> !Kung women provide the majority of the food, spending two to three days a week foraging varying distances from the camp, and are also responsible for child care, gathering wood for fires, carrying water, and cooking. Typical foods they might return with are mongongo nuts, baobab fruits, water roots, bitter melon, or !Gwa berries. Children are left at home to be watched over by those remaining in camp, but nursing children are carried on these foraging trips, adding to the load the !Kung women must carry (Shostak 1981).

As is apparent from this passage, women were able to fulfill many and varied responsibilities while nearly always carrying their nursing children.

BABY CARRYING

One can argue that modern culture is markedly different from that of the hunter-gatherer culture since women today have more diverse responsibilities. The history of baby carrying, however, is very long in the annals of human child-rearing practices. It has only been within the brief period of the past hundred or so years, coinciding with mass urbanization and the development of suburbs, that the tradition of carrying babies and keeping them near their mothers has waned. The culture of distancing newborns from their mothers may be common, but it is a relatively new child-rearing practice.

A century ago, child-rearing experts proclaimed that mothers would spoil their babies by carrying them or providing too much physical affection with hugs and kisses. Without any evidence to support such a preposterous theory, the fear of spoiling babies took root so deeply that it persists to this day. Parents are taught to embrace the culture of keeping their newborns at arm's length even though this is counterintuitive.

Far too many infants, even the tiniest, are often kept strapped into car seats (long after a car ride ends) or strollers when they could easily and safely be carried by their parents. Parents who wish to secure infants more safely to their bodies can use baby carriers, slings, and wraps that are available widely on the Internet. As parents have grown accustomed to keeping infants strapped into car seats and strollers, however, many have become convinced that it is safer not to carry their babies.

This assumption is not necessarily true, as affirmed by a lecture given by Dr. Al Johnson for *PREP: The Course*, a pediatric study program that took place in Costa Mesa from September 11 through 15, 2004. A review of cases involving babies with skull fractures at a major urban hospital showed that 10% of the injuries occurred while the babies were in car seats but not in cars at the time the head trauma occurred. The injured babies were either not buckled properly and fell out of the car seats or they were buckled properly, but the car seats tipped over or fell off an elevated platform like a tabletop.

Irrespective of a baby's need to be carried by her parents, the business sector has come up with an endless array of things that increase the physical distance between parents and even the youngest of babies. The list of items most new parents desire include cribs, strollers, car seats that can fit onto stroller bases, bouncing seats, infant swings, stationary infant seats, play pens, and more. When one becomes enamored of the numerous things one can buy, it may be difficult to perceive how natural it is to carry a baby in one's arms.

For instance, my sister is a wonderful mother who became fascinated with her son's Peg Perego stroller. Although my sister carried her son in a baby carrier in the newborn period, she soon transferred her son to the stroller constantly. She is an artist, and her husband is an industrial designer. Between the two of them, they fell in love with the design and convenience of their son's stroller because it fit everywhere inside and outside their home. At four months of age, the baby was strolled down the hallway inside their apartment.

After witnessing my sister's use of the stroller, I found myself using the stroller for my daughter much more often than I had with my son. Whereas I had generally carried my son, I placed my daughter in her stroller often. Without realizing it, I had become deeply influenced by my sister's love of her stroller. In truth, both my daughter and my nephew were remarkably content in their strollers, and this probably gave my sister and me less incentive to carry our young babies.

In a sense, I was doing what so many other parents appeared to be doing. Using strollers for small babies had become the norm, and I simply followed the trend. It was not until after I read books like Ashley Montagu's *Touching: The Human Significance of the Skin* and Mariana Caplan's *Untouched* that I began to understand the importance of baby carrying. At the risk of sounding like a hypocrite since I did use a stroller often for my daughter, I find it refreshing to see other women carry their babies.

Several years ago, I used to enjoy observing a lissome young mother carrying her baby. I was drawn to watching this dyad whenever I waited to pick up my son from school. It was a pleasure to observe the mother walk purposefully across the school yard to pick up her elder daughter while she carried her adorable little baby. The baby got bigger and bigger, but she was always in her mother's arms, and she looked wonderfully content.

Irrespective of modern parenting trends, a mother's physical availability and proximity are crucial to the well-being of the immature newborn. Every newborn, no matter how large and robust she may be at birth, is actually an immature human being with many needs. The newborn needs to receive the warmth, touch, comfort, and nourishment of her mother's body. The newborn's need for "a womb with a view" is indescribably important since the mother-fetus union that began with pregnancy should not end abruptly with birth simply because a physical separation has occurred.

SATISFACTION OF THE NEWBORN'S NEEDS

Once a newborn emerges from the womb, he is no longer assured the consistent warmth of the womb and the continuous infusion of nutrients from the placenta. Instead, he experiences the new and uncomfortable sensations of cold and hunger. He can urinate as freely as he did in the womb, but he will experience a different sensation on the skin that he has wet. The newborn cannot depend upon the comfort of a small and warm space since he has emerged into an expansive and cold new world outside the womb. The newborn must now negotiate the environment always with the assistance of a person other than himself.

Concomitantly, once the baby is out of the womb, a mother can no longer rely on her body to provide for her baby automatically and without conscious input. Throughout pregnancy, a healthy mother's body undergoes significant hormonal changes in order to accommodate the well-being of the fetus in the womb. Nearly everything that is provided for the fetus does not require a mother's conscious input. This does not mean, however, that pregnancy is a mindless activity.

Indeed, many women make conscientious efforts to improve their health and nutritional status when they become pregnant. They may take vitamin and mineral supplements, improve their diets, and abstain from smoking cigarettes and drinking alcohol. Some women will reduce their stress level because they are aware that the developing fetus may experience similar stress via hormonal influences. On the whole, though, there is not a great deal that most healthy pregnant women need to do to create a healthy womb.

As mentioned earlier, a healthy pregnant woman hardly has to think about the care of her fetus since the physiological changes of pregnancy are all directed hormonally by the conceptus. This is why most healthy pregnant women can proceed with their daily lives without much ado. The amazing simplicity and efficiency of pregnancy, however, may belie the significant changes that childbirth will eventually entail. After an easy pregnancy and childbirth, some parents may even be misled into believing that their lives will not change significantly after a baby's birth.

Perhaps it was because my first childbirth experience was difficult that I felt my life had changed irrevocably. After my son's discharge from the hospital, I felt privileged to provide him with the nurturing that I was unable to offer for the six weeks he was hospitalized. This meant that my days often revolved around breastfeeding him, changing his diaper and clothing, holding him, talking to him, taking him for walks in a baby carrier, and bathing him.

There were times when I would linger in the apartment and wait for my son to awaken from his nap. As I write this, it sounds as if my life was boring and uninspiring. Around that time, my astute six-year-old niece commented that it was tiresome to watch my two-month-old son on videotape for two hours since all he did was sleep and occasionally open his eyes.

It was difficult to relay to others how enjoyable it was to satisfy my son's needs and feel free to take care of him. In truth, I was fulfilling my son's needs as well as my own need to mother him and be there for him. As simple as these mothering activities were, I did not doubt his need for me to be there for him. I was part of my son's existence just as he was part of mine.

My son and I had been as closely united during pregnancy as two human beings could ever be. His birth could not change the union we experienced. His understanding of love was centered on the satisfaction of needs he experienced as a helpless baby. As his mother, I wanted to reply in the best way I could and that was to breastfeed him and be there for him. In other words, as much as my son deserved a "womb with a view," I wanted to be the one to provide that external womb for him.

3

INFANT FORMULA

THE ASSAULT OF THE INFANT FORMULA INDUSTRY

It is commonly assumed that breastfeeding should come naturally to women. It is untrue, however, that a woman will know how to breastfeed her newborn simply because she has been physiologically prepared by pregnancy to breastfeed. Breastfeeding is not instinctive; it is a learned behavior. Exposed constantly to bottle-feeding and rarely to breastfeeding, a great number of women today no longer have much, if any, personal experience with breastfeeding.

Since many women know little about breastfeeding, they may be intimidated or perplexed by the ways in which breastfeeding may be misrepresented to the public. For instance, breastfeeding mothers may be charged with indecency for unintentionally exposing a portion of their breasts to nurse their babies, or they may be expelled from public areas like shopping malls for "lewd" behavior. Additionally, women who promote breastfeeding are frequently accused of being intolerant of those who do not breastfeed.

In the U.S., the American Academy of Pediatrics (AAP) advises exclusive breastfeeding of infants for the first six months of life, which is defined as follows: "…an infant's consumption of human milk with no supplementation of any type (no water, no juice, no nonhuman milk, and no foods) except for vitamins, minerals, and medications" (AAP 2005). For the first six months of life, exclusively breastfed babies have no need for supplementation with infant formula, milk formulations, juice, rice cereal, or any other liquids or solids.

In other words, healthy babies need to drink only breast milk for the entire first six months of life. Breastfeeding is species-specific, cost effective, and provides youngsters the best available protection from disease. Regrettably, few families are cognizant of the tremendous benefits of breastfeeding.

Much of the ignorance surrounding breastfeeding's benefits is a consequence of the miseducation that infant formula advertisements present to the general public. The infant formula industry spends millions of dollars annually to promote the sale of infant formula. Advertisements on television and in magazines praise the supposed normalcy and the convenience of using infant formula. The Lifetime cable television channel and morning television talk shows, which are geared toward female audiences, air infant formula commercials frequently. The primary purpose of these ads is to encourage infant formula consumption, and there is little doubt that parents are influenced strongly to use infant formula instead of breastfeeding.

In addition, the infant formula industry underwrites various freebies that are offered frequently to new mothers. This means that new mothers may leave hospitals with complimentary bottles of ready-to-use infant formula, coupons for infant formula, and various knick-knacks that are emblazoned with the brand names of infant formula. Once they arrive home, new mothers may receive unsolicited mailings of infant formula coupons because their names and addresses have been released to the infant formula companies by hospitals.

As a pregnant pediatrician, I once received a complimentary gift basket from an infant formula sales representative. I examined the basket's contents and realized that it was not a personal gift but a big push for this sales representative's brand of infant formula. Every item in the basket, including electrical outlet plugs and pacifiers, had the infant formula manufacturer imprint on it.

During my tenure as a practicing pediatrician, this sales representative had always been more courteous and respectful than a sales representative of another major brand of formula. The latter had nurtured a long-time relationship with my more established colleague, and his brand of infant formula was more visible in our office. Even so, when parents asked me which formula I would recommend, I tended to endorse the product offered by the friendlier sales representative. Indubitably, pediatricians are swayed to recommend infant formula products, and the reasoning behind such support may be completely unscientific and biased by personal sentiments, such as preferring one sales representative over another.

THE POWERFUL INFANT FORMULA INDUSTRY

The underlying message behind infant formula advertising campaigns and the sales techniques of the industry's various sales representatives is that a baby needs a bottle in his mouth. Currently, the most popular image of babyhood is the baby bottle, which is a tangible object that advertisers can use to sell profitable products such as infant formula. In contrast, breastfeeding is not marketed since the advertising industry cannot earn money from its promotion. There is no concrete product to sell to consumers since human milk cannot be manufactured in factories and sold in containers.

Infant formula, in contrast, is most certainly a product that can be sold. This is, in effect, why the infant formula industry began to treat infant formula as a food product in the late 1980s. Manufacturers of infant formula started to offer their products directly to the general public with advertisements and promotions. The industry argued that marketing infant formula was no different from promoting the sale of any other beverage.

The move to advertise to the general public ended a long-standing tradition of permitting only doctors to recommend the use of specific brands of infant formula to patients. Although the American Academy of Pediatrics (AAP) objected, it did not make strenuous efforts to thwart the infant formula industry's plan to pitch sales directly to the general public. Today, the television commercials and magazine advertisements that promote the use of infant formula are part of modern culture.

The infant formula industry, which consists of giant pharmaceutical and food conglomerates, uses sales techniques that are not dissimilar from those used by the powerful tobacco industry. For example, the tobacco industry was able to convince millions of citizens to smoke cigarettes even as the medical community produced evidence of the harm that cigarette smoking caused. Similarly, the infant formula industry manipulates the dissemination of information regarding infant feeding so that consumers perceive infant formula to be a convenient, nutritious, and benign product.

The infant formula industry provides most of the monetary grants and funds for scientific research related to infant feeding, including studies of breastfeeding. The infant formula manufacturers also distribute their own written literature about breastfeeding to the general public through physicians' offices, primarily those of obstetricians, family physicians, and pediatricians. The industry is commanding enough, through connected and well-paid lobbyists, that it can influence child health initiatives and policies created or supported by the U.S. government.

For instance, in the fall of 2003, the U.S. Department of Health and Human Services planned to initiate an educational pro-breastfeeding public service campaign (Ross and Rackmill 2004). The information to be aired, however, was altered significantly after the infant formula industry lobbied strongly against the campaign. The industry's lobbyists assessed the ads to be unscientific and too biased against infant formula. Evidently, the infant formula industry did not trust the scientific data that revealed that non-breastfed infants face a 20 percent higher risk of death in the first year of life and that they have a higher risk of infections and cancer. The AAP physicians who helped to create the ads, including pediatrician and breastfeeding advocate Lawrence Gartner, were disappointed that the AAP did not support the original public service campaign.

Such interference with breastfeeding education is not benign since the industry promotes the multi-billion dollar yearly sale of infant formula and the wholesale separation of mother from infant. Routinely, commercial and print advertisements showcase pretty actresses cuddling and feeding infant formula in bottles to adorable babies. These ads are insidious since they glorify the image of mother-infant bonding while they dismiss the importance of breastfeeding in enhancing healthy mother-infant bonding. The ads appear to reveal the beauty of mother-infant bonding, but the substance of the bonding seems to arise from the use of infant formula and definitely not from breastfeeding.

THE MILK IN INFANT FORMULA

Parents should wonder about the source of the cow's milk that eventually becomes infant formula. Although cow's milk should be reserved for nursing calves, the docility of cows makes them an easily accessible and abundant source of milk. Most milk is no longer collected by farmers for individual family use; instead, milk is produced commercially so that milk products may be distributed widely.

The milk that is offered to the general public and used to manufacture infant formula is extracted from dairy cows that may have been exposed to the following: a) pesticides, fungicides, and chemical fertilizers (from the grains cows are given to eat since most have no access to grass, which should be their normal and primary source of food); b) growth hormone (that may be injected into cows every other week so that there will be a 10% increase in milk production); c) and antibiotics to treat stomach or liver infections that may arise since cows have difficulty digesting grains, as well as udder infections that may result from administration of growth hormone. In effect, most dairy cows are not raised to produce nutritious milk for their nursing calves but to produce copious amounts of milk rapidly and perhaps artificially for commercial distribution.

Parents may feel reassured that organic infant formula is a better option than regular infant formula. They might not feel as confident after they read Michael Pollan's article, entitled "Behind the Organic-Industrial Complex," in the May 12, 2001 of the *New York Times Magazine*. Pollan investigates the origins of costlier and ostensibly healthier organic milk that is sold nationwide by Horizon, a public company that states on its cartons that it distributes milk from over 3,000 "family farms." Pollan comments wryly that some of these farms may actually be "factory farms" where "thousands of cows that never encounter a blade of grass spend their days confined to a fenced dry lot, eating (certified organic) grain and tethered to milking machines three times a day."

Pollan learns from a local dairyman that milk from these factory farms is ultra-pasteurized, which means that the milk is treated at high temperature to ensure sterility and prolonged freshness. Ultra-pasteurization is a process that kills active enzymes and vitamins that are normally found in raw milk or regularly pasteurized milk. Thus, organic milk-based infant formula may be free of fertilizers, pesticides, antibiotics, and hormones. It does not necessarily mean, however, that organic milk-based infant formula is more nutritious than regular infant formula.

Cow's milk may be the primary ingredient for most brands of infant formula, but parents should also be concerned about the soybeans that are used to create popular soy-based infant formula. Soybeans have become a major worldwide crop, and they are usually grown with chemical fertilizers, pesticides, and fungicides. Therefore, it is possible that infant formula that is based upon soy milk may contain traces of fertilizers, pesticides, and fungicides. Clearly, parents should be better informed about the source of the milk that is used to manufacture infant formula since infants are either breastfed or fed infant formula for the first twelve months of life.

WHAT IS INFANT FORMULA?

Infant formula is produced in factories where fixed recipes are used to add various components together exactly the same way every time. Machines process cow's milk or soy milk to create a liquid or powder product that is pasteurized and preserved in order to assure a long shelf life. The purpose of a long shelf life is not for the benefit of a baby's health but for the profit of an industry that does not need to concern itself with the immediate freshness of its products. This means that the average infant formula powdered product expires three years after its original production date.

Regardless of its age but before its expiration date, infant formula can be dispensed directly from a can or reconstituted by adding water to concentrated liquid or powder. In other words, by the time a baby ingests infant formula it is a dead product that is devoid of life. Infant formula is a highly processed and adulterated food, and it is the primary source of nourishment for an inordinately high percentage of healthy young babies.

In contrast, breast milk is a dynamic and living liquid that changes constantly according to the baby's needs. It is produced on demand and freshly for a specific baby since every woman's breast milk is unique. Despite the huge differences in quality between breast milk and infant formula, nevertheless, the majority of healthy young babies continue to receive the nourishment of dead fluid from another species or a plant source for the greater part of or the entire first year of life.

It is curious to note that in a society whose citizens' tastes have become universally refined, few individuals bother to differentiate the quality of infant formula from that of breast milk. As aware as some parents may be of the contents of infant formula, many others may be uninformed. A quick search of Netgrocer.com on the Internet yields the following ingredient list for Similac with Iron Infant Formula in the Ready to Use liquid form:

WATER
NONFAT MILK
LACTOSE
HIGH-OLEIC SAFFLOWER OIL
COCONUT OIL
SOY OIL
WHEY PROTEIN CONCENTRATE
LESS THAN 0.5 PERCENT OF:

CALCIUM CARBONATE, POTASSIUM CITRATE, MAGNESIUM CHLORIDE, POTASSIUM CHLORIDE, SODIUM CHLORIDE, FERROUS SULFATE, ZINC SULFATE, MONO-AND DIGLYCERIDES, SOY LECITHIN, CARRAGEENAN, TAURINE, INOSITOL, CUPRIC SULFATE, MANGANESE SULFATE, SODIUM SELENATE, CHOLINE BITARTRATE, ASCORBIC

> ACID, ALPHA-TOCOPHERYL ACETATE, NIACINAMIDE, CALCIUM PANTOTHENATE, VITAMIN A PALMITATE, THIAMINE CHLORIDE HYDROCHLORIDE, RIBOFLAVIN, PYRIDOXINE HYDROCHLORIDE, BETA-CAROTENE, FOLIC ACID, PHYLLOQUINONE, BIOTIN, VITAMIN D3, CYANOCOBALAMIN, AND NUCLEOTIDES (ADENOSINE 5'-MONOPHOSPHATE, CYTIDINE 5'-MONOPHOSPHATE, DISODIUM GUANOSINE 5'-MONOPHOSPHATE, DISODIUM URIDINE 5'-MONOPHOSPHATE).

This popular brand of infant formula contains less than 40 ingredients whereas breast milk contains more than 200 ingredients. The absence of over 160 ingredients in infant formula is a huge discrepancy that is not remarked upon by either infant formula manufacturers or the majority of health practitioners.

The Food and Drug Administration (FDA), which oversees the production of human milk substitutes to the general public, sets standards that are implausibly limited. Current FDA regulations require minimum amounts of 29 nutrients and maximum amounts of nine of these nutrients in infant formula (Food and Drug Administration 2003). The disparity between a minimum of 29 ingredients in infant formula and over 200 naturally occurring substances in human milk is tremendous but apparently readily overlooked.

It may be possible to understand the widespread and fairly blind acceptance of processed infant formula in a decade like the 1950s when Velveeta cheese, Wonder bread, and instant coffee were staples in most American kitchens. By the turn of the twenty-first century, however, consumers had already witnessed the burgeoning growth and development of farmers markets, the natural food industry, as well as organic and sustainable farming. Although the general public still enjoys the convenience of eating processed foods, more people are looking for higher quality in the foods they choose to consume.

Consumers today, in fact, are willing to pay a premium price for fresher and more natural foods. As consumers have become better educated, they have become more interested in the quality of the foods they eat. Increasingly, foods are scrutinized for artificial preservatives, additives, and types of sugars and fats. Consumers also check produce for freshness, and they may discriminate against buying any that have been grown with pesticides or chemical fertilizers. In response to the growing interest and demand for fresher and more natural foods, the organic and sustainable food markets continue to expand in increasing numbers and types of grocery stores and food purveyors.

Even as more consumers seek higher quality in food for adults and children, however, the same cannot be said of what is offered to young babies in the form of infant formula. It is highly doubtful that health-conscious adults would consume infant formula daily as their primary source of nourishment for one year. Paradoxically, even highly educated food consumers may not think twice about feeding their babies infant formula.

One cannot help but conclude that most consumers are not examining carefully enough the ingredient list of infant formula. Undoubtedly, this is because parents do not feel the need to question the contents or safety of infant formula. In a sense, they may waive their responsibility to think for themselves because they trust the medical community and the U.S. government to provide their babies with safe infant formula. Regrettably, this is the type of misinformed thinking that led millions of Americans to trust the tobacco industry's advertisements that citizens could enjoy smoking cigarettes while appearing to maintain excellent health.

The hazards of cigarette smoking, as noted on the Surgeon General's warning that has been printed on cigarette boxes since 1964, were not taken seriously by most citizens or even the U.S. government. In fact, the government promoted cigarette smoking in the military for decades through the rationing of cigarettes as rewards. It was not until 1975 that the U.S. government stopped distributing cigarettes in K-rations and C-rations to soldiers and sailors (CDC 2004b). Unfortunately, the culture of cigarette smoking remains pervasive in the military, and the consequences are on display at the nation's Veterans Administration hospitals, in which many thousands of veterans suffer from emphysema and diseases related to cigarette smoking.

It should also be noted that many physicians did not take an active role in discouraging patients from smoking cigarettes until the recent past. As mentioned earlier, pregnant women were smoking cigarettes with their physicians' knowledge even in the mid-1970s. The pervasive assumption was that citizens were informed enough to decide whether or not to smoke cigarettes, irrespective of advertisements, physician advice, and cultural influences.

It can be argued that health concerns about cigarette smoking do not dissuade addicted smokers from ceasing to smoke cigarettes. Economist Paul Krugman points out in a *New York Times* column on July 8, 2005, however, that the educational campaign to alert the public about the hazards of cigarette smoking has succeeded in decreasing U.S. cigarette consumption per capita by more than 50 percent since the 1960s. When more citizens understood how harmful cigarette smoking was to smokers as well as those in their immediate environment, many people stopped smoking or never started smoking at all.

The reality is that although the general public implicitly understood the power of the tobacco industry, many citizens were unaware of the duplicitous ways in which the tobacco industry sought to deceive citizens. As recently as the mid-1990s, the CEOs of the major tobacco corporations were brazen enough to testify under oath and before Congress that they did not believe that nicotine was addictive. It will become similarly manifest in the near future that the American public's trust in the safety of infant formula as it is presented by the infant formula industry and the U.S. government was short-sighted and in poor judgment.

CONTAMINATED INFANT FORMULA

The repeated claim that the use of infant formula is healthful is curious and suspect, particularly when there are serious problems associated with the manufacture of infant formula. Over a ten-year period between 1983–1993, "formula was recalled twenty-two times due to safety problems, well over half from instances where the product would cause death or serious health consequences, in some cases, irreversible" (Baumslag and Michels 1995, 103).

Jeff McDonald reports in the November 5, 2002, issue of the *San Diego Tribune* that Wyeth Nutritionals, a division of conglomerate American Home Products and a major infant formula manufacturer, recalled 1.5 million cans of powdered infant formula that were sold under 12 different brand names, including Baby Basics, CVS, Healthy Baby, Safeway Select, and Walgreens. The formula may have been contaminated with the bacterium *Enterobacter sakazakii*, which is food-borne and may cause sepsis (widespread infection through the bloodstream), meningitis, or severe gastrointestinal infections. The formula was manufactured between July and September 2002 and was stamped with an expiration date between July and September 2005. If this formula had not been recalled, the bacteria would have had a chance to grow and reproduce for three years or even longer since some grocers and consumers ignore expiration dates.

A report issued by the Canadian government notes that *Enterobacter sakazakii* is a frequent bacterial contaminant of powdered infant formula, and the reported case-fatality rate varies from 40 to 80 percent among neonates diagnosed with this severe infection (Health Canada 2002). The report also mentions that there have been outbreaks of *E. sakazakii* in Neonatal Intensive Care Units all over the world, including England, the Netherlands, the U.S., and Greece. The Canadian government advises health professionals to avoid feeding newborns with reconstituted powdered infant formula, and they recommend instead Ready to Use or concentrated liquid infant formula.

The World Health Organization (WHO) in May 2005 recommended a resolution that would require the placement of a health warning label on powdered infant formula products. A thorough review of available scientific information concluded the following: "...intrinsic contamination of powdered infant formula with *E. sakazakii* and *Salmonella* has been a cause of infection and illness in infants, including severe disease which can lead to serious developmental sequelae and death" (WHO 2005). The review noted that the manufacture of powdered infant formula does not include a step in which bacteria such as *E. sakazakii* and *Salmonella* are killed. The fundamental problem is that powdered infant formula is not a sterile product. Additionally, powdered infant formula may be tested for bacterial contamination after its manufacture, but the tests are currently for coliform bacteria, like *E. Coli*, and not *Enterobacter.*

There is evidence that powdered infant formula that has been contaminated with one microorganism can cause infection. As mentioned earlier, the fact that expiration dates for powdered infant formula is set for three years after its production date gives contaminants an inordinately long period of time to reproduce. The bacterial contamination of infant formula products has been occurring for decades, but few parents are aware that powdered infant formula is not even sterilized. Why would any parent assume that infant formula is not sterilized? If parents were aware of this risk, they would at least have the option of using liquid infant formula preparations that undergo a bactericidal step during its manufacture.

INEXCUSABLE DEFENSE OF THE INFANT FORMULA INDUSTRY

The WHO resolution is important since there are currently millions of infants worldwide that are fed powdered infant formula. Even so, the U.S. media did not publicize news of the proposed WHO resolution. This is unfortunate since the general public needs to be informed of the potential risks associated with the use of infant formula. It is an egregious oversight on the part of the media to ignore the significance of the WHO resolution.

As an individual who reads two newspapers daily and peruses news on the Internet, I did not learn of the WHO resolution until I read Charlotte Allen's critical commentary in the June 26, 2005, issue of the *Los Angeles Times*. Her commentary, entitled "When Mother's Milk is Just Not Good Enough" was published one month after the WHO resolution was made public. In her commentary, Charlotte Allen expresses disdain for the WHO resolution, and she defends the infant formula industry.

Allen offers the following typical pronouncement on the safety of infant formula: "The Food and Drug Administration has recognized that infant formula from reputable companies, manufactured under stringent government specifications, is perfectly safe and nutritious, provided that precautions are taken against stray bacterial contaminants." She writes this even though WHO researchers found that powdered infant formula is not sterilized during its manufacture, and the infant formula industry is fully aware of this manufacturing omission.

Allen also dislikes the WHO recommendation that children be breastfed for at least two years and derides such practices as being more attuned to the lifestyles of those in a "hippie commune." Inexplicably and inexcusably, she actually defends Nestlé's attempts to popularize the use of infant formula in Africa in the 1970s. Poor women in Africa could not afford infant formula, and many had no access to clean water. Once these poverty stricken women stopped breastfeeding after using free samples of infant formula, they could only continue to use infant formula. Many women were found to be watering down the infant formula in order to make it last longer. Meanwhile, their babies were malnourished and ill with infections they would have been protected from had they been breastfed.

UNICEF (2005) estimates that breastfeeding could save the lives of approximately 1.3 million babies annually. Allen, however, can claim that breastfeeding advocates are simply upset that infant formula manufacturers earn money. She writes, "Big corporations make—horrors—profits on formula sales, so they must be duly demonized." Such a facile interpretation of breastfeeding advocacy is worrisome and demeaning to the numerous non-profit worldwide organizations, including La Leche League (which Allen targets specifically), that work to enhance the well-being and health of children. Even though the deaths of 1.3 million babies could be averted through the promotion of breastfeeding, Allen disparages efforts to encourage women to breastfeed. Apparently, Allen is not interested in understanding the true costs associated with the use of infant formula.

THE COST OF INFANT FORMULA

Many parents will choose to use infant formula, but some may underestimate the costs of using it. A competitive price of $4.99 appeared in May 2005 on Netgrocer.com on the Internet for a 13-fluid ounce can of Similac infant formula with iron in concentrated liquid form. This means that feeding a baby 26 ounces of liquid infant formula with iron costs $4.99 and the following: a) the time and gasoline needed to drive to and from the grocery store, b) the cost of using and washing bottles and nipples, c) the gas or electricity and water used to boil and clean the bottles and nipples, and d) the cost of bottled water that many parents use to dilute concentrated liquid formula or to reconstitute powdered formula. Overall, the overt cost of using infant formula as a form of infant feeding accumulates.

As a pediatrician, I had access to complimentary infant formula from an infant formula sales representative who visited my pediatric office regularly. After my son's birth, she sent me a case of canned infant formula. I gave it to a friend who had not realized how costly infant formula would be.

Another friend of mine decided against breastfeeding because she thought that her seven-year-old daughter was jealous of her nursing baby sister. Choosing infant formula proved to be disastrous since her infant turned out to be allergic to nearly all infant formulas. The baby was ultimately able to tolerate only a costly infant formula that contained predigested protein. The cost of the prohibitively expensive protein hydrosylate formula was an unexpected burden at a time when the family was experiencing significant financial troubles.

Parents may choose not to breastfeed without pondering seriously the financial cost of using infant formula. There are also numerous hidden costs associated with the use of infant formula. In a nation that does not provide universal health coverage for young children, it would be appropriate to encourage mothers to offer young children the best possible health protection early in life, which is breastfeeding. Breastfed babies experience a far lower incidence of childhood infectious illnesses even when they are placed in day care. On the whole, breastfed children experience better health; less pain and suffering with illnesses; and fewer visits to doctors' offices, hospitalizations, and medication and prescription bills.

Regrettably, the general public continues to receive a barrage of misleading information from the infant formula industry and unhelpful guidance from the medical community. Obstetricians often do not stress the importance of breastfeeding to pregnant women because they trust women's ability to make independent decisions about infant feeding. This is hardly possible, however, when women are bombarded with infant formula ads from the media, and they receive insufficiently accurate information about breastfeeding from physicians.

For instance, obstetricians distribute free and seemingly unbiased prenatal literature to pregnant women. The ostensibly objective infant feeding literature, unbeknownst to many prospective parents, is written by infant formula manufacturers. Consequently, the message from the literature is almost always that infant formula is a good substitute for breastfeeding. The lack of guidance from obstetricians, combined with the dissemination of infant formula-biased literature about infant feeding, makes many obstetricians complicit in the failure to enhance greater understanding of breastfeeding's significance.

Whereas obstetricians may promote the use of infant formula indirectly, family physicians and pediatricians often endorse the practice overtly. Pediatric offices, for instance, may be decorated with posters that appeal to young children and contain the logos of various infant formula brands; magazine racks may be filled with parenting magazines that contain numerous infant formula advertisements; and various knick-knacks all over the examining rooms and the waiting room, like electrical outlet plugs or even magazine racks, may advertise infant formula. The offices of family physicians and pediatricians are also generally well-stocked with infant formula samples that can be distributed for free to patients. The consequence of using these free samples is that parents will run out of them, so they will need to buy more infant formula on their own.

Since primary care health practitioners are supposed to ensure babies' good health by advocating preventive measures, it only makes sense that they should promote breastfeeding. Breastfeeding, after all, is the ideal preventive measure that best ensures good health for mothers and infants. By all appearances, though, the economics of selling infant formula overpowers the economics of promoting good health.

THE IRREPLACEABLE NATURE OF BREAST MILK

Health writer Janis Graham interviewed William MacLean, Jr., vice president of pediatric research and development at Ross Products, a division of the pharmaceutical giant Abbott Laboratories and the maker of Similac brand of infant formula. MacLean admits the following to Graham (1995, 102): "We will never be able to put breast milk in a can. In the strict sense, formulas are no longer made to duplicate breast milk. They're made to imitate the way breast milk is *metabolized* by babies." In other words, as Janis Graham notes in her article, the infant formula industry does not even attempt to duplicate the contents of breast milk.

Instead, the industry strives to get infant formula to break down to offer nutrients in quantities similar to that offered by breast milk. For example, because 49 percent of the iron in breast milk is absorbed efficiently, the iron content of breast milk is low (Baumslag and Michels 1995, 86). In contrast, only four percent of the iron in infant formula is absorbed, so the iron content of infant formula must be much higher. Hence, there are numerous iron-fortified infant formulas whose iron content is much higher than that of breast milk.

This significant difference between breast milk and infant formula, however, is not publicized. Instead, the infant formula industry encourages the general public and health practitioners to dismiss such discrepancies. Intriguingly, advertisements are effective enough to convince the general public and health practitioners that infant formula is not dissimilar from breast milk. Consequently, consumers are unaware of the tremendous differences between breast milk and infant formula. (See Appendix A to learn more about the incomparable contents of breast milk.)

Infant formula, however, is either missing or deficient in ingredients that are supplied naturally in breast milk. For instance, the amino acid tryptophan is present in great concentration in colostrum (the secretions the breasts yield in the early newborn period), and it is found in breast milk. In contrast, the bioavailability of tryptophan in milk-based infant formulas is lower than that of tryptophan found naturally in breast milk.

One study noted that infant formulas supplied in dried powder form had from a little over one-half to a little over two-thirds of bioavailable tryptophan as compared to breast milk (Sarwar and Botting 1999). Liquid concentrate had less bioavailable tryptophan than the dried powder form of infant formula, which is unfortunate since as mentioned earlier powdered infant formula has a higher risk of bacterial contamination than liquid formula. Supplementation of liquid concentrate with tryptophan resulted in elevated levels of tryptophan in the plasma and brain, as well as increased levels of serotonin in the brain. The authors of the study concluded that more research is needed to investigate the influence that tryptophan supplementation to infant formula would have upon infants' sleep and neurobehavioral development.

Tryptophan is essential for the production of serotonin, an important chemical in the brain that regulates emotion and produces a state of calm and well-being. Numerous studies have shown that imbalances in the level of serotonin can trigger depression. As a result, the most prevalent therapeutic approach to the treatment of depression involves medication with substances that are believed to regulate levels of serotonin, like Serotonin Reuptake Inhibitors (SSRIs) such as Prozac, Paxil, or Zoloft.

Serious concerns have been raised in recent years, however, about the significant risks associated with the use of SSRIs in young children and adolescents. It appears that officials of the Food and Drug Administration (FDA) were aware of an increase in suicidal thoughts and behaviors linked to the use of SSRIs in children as early as March 1996, but the agency took no action until 2003 (Rosack 2004). As of late 2004, the FDA requires pharmaceutical companies to add to all anti-depressants "black box" warnings, which state that "these medications may cause suicidal thoughts and/or behavior in some children and adolescents" (Gurian 2004).

Tragically, some children who were prescribed these medications have already taken their own lives. These children's parents are lobbying strenuously for greater oversight of SSRI prescribing practices. In the meantime, other parents attribute their children's more stable mental health status to successful treatment with SSRIs. In light of the ongoing concerns about prescribing anti-depressants to youngsters, it is apparent that there are far too many mentally ill children and adolescents who have problems with serotonin regulation in their brains.

The reality is that tryptophan deficiency in infant formula is a glaring oversight since the correlation between abnormalities in serotonin regulation and depression has been known for decades. Research should be performed to examine the relationship between the widespread use of infant formula that is deficient in tryptophan, an important serotonin precursor, and the increased prevalence of depression and mental illness among children and adolescents. The millions of infants who drink infant formula deserve a better and more healthful product.

BETTER INFANT FORMULA?

Despite the fact that infant formula contains inadequate amounts of key ingredients for healthy human development, the infant formula manufacturers are not dissuaded. They continue to advertise their products constantly to the public despite the abundant research that demonstrates the superiority of breastfeeding. Industry executives understand that bottle-feeding has become a cultural norm and that it will take many years before the general public becomes aware of the importance of breastfeeding. In the meantime, by adding a few ingredients to infant formula, the industry feels free to promote infant formula products that it claims are now more comparable to breast milk.

For example, in 2001 the Food and Drug Administration (FDA) allowed the sale of infant formulas that has been fortified with two fatty acids that are found naturally in breast milk. The fatty acids are an omega-3 fatty acid, DHA (docosahexaenoic acid), and an omega-6 fatty acid, ARA (arachidonic acid). DHA has been found to be necessary for brain development and for visual acuity (Baumslag and Michels 1995, 84). The addition of ARA to infant formula was hypothesized to improve growth of preterms in the first year of life after supplementation with DHA and another omega-3-fatty acid appeared to result in lower total growth of infants (Brenna 2004). Infant formulas that are fortified with DHA and ARA are touted as being more like breast milk.

Most consumers are not aware, however, that the recent addition of DHA and ARA supplements to some infant formula preparations was *permitted but not approved* by the FDA. Before the FDA grants approval for the sale of DHA and ARA supplemented formula, it wants to study the long-term benefits and risks associated with its use (Food and Drug Administration 2003). The FDA permitted the sale of this supplemented infant formula because of consumer demand and the lobbying efforts of infant formula manufacturers. In other words, babies who currently drink infant formula supplemented with DHA and ARA are part of an ongoing experiment.

It should be noted that the supplemental fatty acids that are added to infant formula are not species-specific for human babies. Breast milk provides DHA and ARA that are created for human infants. Although different sources of DHA and ARA are available, most notably fish oil, the FDA has approved for use in infant formula only DHA that has been extracted from unicellular algae cultured in bioreactors and ARA extracted from a fungus (Brenna 2003).

Lactation consultant Marsha Walker (2004) offers some insight into potential problems associated with the use of infant formula that has been supplemented with DHA and ARA. She cites the possible side effects of explosive, watery diarrhea that may interfere with adequate fat and vitamin absorption; the possible contribution of these oils to the growing epidemic of obesity in the U.S.; the potential harm of the fungal source of ARA acting as a pathogen in babies with compromised immune systems; and evidence of liver damage in rat experiments. Although infant formulas that are fortified with DHA and ARA are purported to be more like breast milk, albeit at a 10 to 15 percent price higher than that of conventional infant formula, the fact remains that breast milk cannot be duplicated and attempts to even try to offer an adequate replacement are grossly insufficient.

In comparison, by passing breast milk on to her young child, a mother can offer her child the best nourishment at the lowest price possible. Breast milk is a product free of cost, so it is troubling that as cost-conscious as American consumers have become, many cannot perceive the economic advantages of breastfeeding. The production and secretion of breast milk require none of the following: packaging, shipping, fear of contamination from incorrect formulations or machinery breakdown, expiration dates (except when expressed and stored), or midnight runs to the store for insufficient milk. Breast milk is an extraordinarily economic and efficient product.

THE CULTURE OF BOTTLE-FEEDING

Since modern Western culture embraces bottle-feeding, it is often difficult for parents to obtain helpful information about breastfeeding. In the majority of parenting books, breastfeeding is discussed cursorily and always with the added caveat that infant formula is a good substitute for women who cannot or do not wish to breastfeed. Rather than address the problem of why women cannot or will not breastfeed, most parenting books simply acknowledge the fact that many women will choose not to breastfeed.

One may understand why women chose not to breastfeed back in the 1950s since physicians proclaimed openly the superiority of bottle-feeding and actively discouraged breastfeeding. A friend pointed out to me that women of our mothers' generation were frequently advised that breastfeeding was harmful to their babies. Some women, like my friend's mother, were even prescribed a medication to dry up their milk.

Such drugs like the dopamine agonist, Bromocriptine, suppress lactation by inhibiting the release of prolactin from the pituitary gland. One study showed that the use of Bromocriptine was associated with an increased risk of hypertension in women (Watson et al. 1989). Fortunately, Bromocriptine is no longer prescribed by physicians since its use may also be associated with potential risks such as strokes, seizures, and myocardial infarctions (Drugs.com 1997).

According to breastfeeding researcher Dr. Ruth Lawrence at the University of Rochester, there is a low incidence of pain experienced by women who choose not to breastfeed (Stehlin 1990). The experience of discomfort associated with breast swelling in the absence of breastfeeding can be relieved with over-the-counter analgesics like acetaminophen or ice packs. Clearly, women in the past should not have been prescribed potentially harmful drugs like Bromocriptine since there are no apparent risks associated with ending lactation naturally.

Throughout human history, breastfeeding has not always been possible for a diverse group of people. Hence, there has always been a need for safe and nourishing alternatives to breastfeeding. A small minority of women may face death unexpectedly, and some may be ill. Some women may experience extraordinary difficulty with breastfeeding. Even among women who seek the expert assistance of lactation consultants, some find that breastfeeding is too difficult. Also, there will always be women who simply do not wish to breastfeed for profoundly personal reasons. My sister reminded me recently that there are individuals who are repelled by the mere thought of breastfeeding. Thus, the use of infant formula is important for women who choose not to breastfeed.

Infant formula is equally essential for families in which newborns and babies are reared in the absence of the children's biological mothers. Every day, babies are sadly abandoned, happily adopted, or cared for primarily by relatives or non-maternal caregivers. In all these various cases, infant formula provides caregivers with an invaluable alternative to breastfeeding that is deemed to be safe by most health practitioners. For obvious reasons, then, infant formula should be manufactured for the unusual cases in which mothers are unavailable to breastfeed.

As mentioned earlier, however, the infant formula industry has succeeded in turning infant formula into a food item that is readily available to the general public. Like most food items, infant formula is advertised frequently, and discount coupons are available in grocery store flyers. Infant formula can be purchased at wholesale outlets like Costco as well as via the Internet from purveyors like Amazon.com. The widespread availability of infant formula assures that it is no longer used as a last resort for babies who absolutely cannot be breastfed.

Many healthy women offer infant formula to their healthy babies without thinking twice since bottle-feeding is a cultural norm. Even women who understand the benefits of breastfeeding will supplement with infant formula because of the convenience it purports to provide. In light of the superior benefits of breastfeeding to infant and maternal health, though, it is surprising how many women trust that infant formula is fine for their babies. In stark contrast to a hundred years ago when few babies were fed infant formula, millions of babies are now fed infant formula.

THE INCONVENIENCE OF BOTTLE-FEEDING

Although women have varying reasons for choosing to bottle-feed, some women learn only after they stop breastfeeding that the use of infant formula is not that simple. For instance, childbirth educator Susan McCutcheon felt she was breastfeeding her first baby constantly (1996, 226–228). She switched to infant formula and learned that the baby was drinking formula just as frequently. She realized after she stopped breastfeeding that she would have preferred to keep struggling with breastfeeding instead of worrying about running out of infant formula or trying to assuage a hungry baby.

A friend of mine had a similar realization after she stopped breastfeeding her first child. He seemed to spit up constantly after nursing, so she switched to infant formula when he was six months old. She found afterward that preparing infant formula instead of having a breast available was more work than she had envisioned. She wound up breastfeeding her second child for eighteen months.

Some parents, like my friend, may be perturbed by the frequency with which some breastfed babies may spit up. Pediatric gastroenterologist Dr. Michael J. Nowicki notes, however, that breastfed babies spit up for a good teleological reason. He gave a lecture for *PREP: The Course*, a pediatric study program that was held in Costa Mesa from September 11 through 15, 2004. Breast milk, Dr. Nowicki comments, is far more than oral nutrition: it contains numerous active anti-inflammatory substances that coat the back of the throat when babies spit up. The spit up milk acts to protect the entire ear, nose, throat region from infection and decreases babies' risk of getting ear and sinus infections.

This important perspective on spitting up is not widely known, however, and many parents may be frustrated if their breastfed babies tend to spit up. With all the advertisements of the convenience of using infant formula, parents receive the impression that bottle-feeding is easier than breastfeeding. Contrary to the pronouncements of advertisements, nevertheless, bottle-feeding is hardly convenient.

Consider the following directions that accompany Similac with iron concentrated liquid infant formula:

Directions:

1. Boil bottles, nipples and rings for 5 minutes, then cool.

2. Heat water for formula to a rolling boil, then cool.

3. Rinse can lid and shake very well. Open with a clean punch-type opener.

4. Pour equal amounts of formula and water into bottle (or cup). Attach a nipple, shake very well, test temperature and feed.

5. Throw away formula remaining in bottle (or cup) after feeding.

Storage: Mixed formula in bottles not used immediately and open can (covered) should be stored in refrigerator. Use within 48 hours. Do not store unopened cans at extreme temperatures.

These directions demonstrate clearly the inconvenience of using infant formula, which involves a great deal of preparation and a significant amount of waste since residual formula after a feeding is supposed to be discarded. Even so, parents trust the contention of advertisements that proclaim the convenience of using infant formula.

DISREGARDING THE GOLD STANDARD OF INFANT FEEDING

In early 2005 the American Academy of Pediatrics (AAP) issued a policy statement that strongly encourages women to breastfeed, and it stated definitively that artificial substitutes differ markedly from breast milk. Included in the AAP policy statement was the following important information:

> Extensive research using improved epidemiologic methods and modern laboratory techniques documents diverse and compelling advantages for infants, mothers, families, and society from breastfeeding and use of human milk for infant feeding. These advantages include health, nutritional, immunologic, developmental, psychologic, social, economic, and environmental benefits.... Human milk is species-specific, and all substitute feeding preparations differ markedly from it, making human milk uniquely superior for infant feeding. Exclusive breastfeeding is the reference or normative model against which all alternative feeding methods must be measured with regard to growth, health, development, and all other short-and long-term outcomes (AAP 2005).

The policy statement affirms that there is no comparison between breastfeeding and infant formula feeding when it comes to disease prevention and mitigation: breastfeeding is the gold standard when it comes to high standards for good infant health.

The infant formula industry is well aware of the AAP's position on breastfeeding. It nevertheless continues to wage its clever war against breastfeeding and mother-infant bonding without acknowledging the risks that are being taken with the health of babies and mothers. Makers of infant formula are aware that their products can never emulate breast milk, but this does not deter them from wording their literature so as to exploit any possible resemblance infant formula may have to breast milk.

Ross Products, the maker of Similac brand of infant formula products, offers the following highlighted statement on their Web site about an infant formula product that contains nucleotides, which are substances found naturally in breast milk: "Similac Advance can help develop both your baby's immune system and brain like breast milk" (Similac 2005). Immediately below it, in smaller italicized letters, Ross Products adds the following statement: "The clinical study showed immune cell development like breast milk. Whether this development provides immune protection like breast milk has not been shown. Breast milk also contains antibodies not found in infant formulas that are important for a baby's immune protection" (Similac 2005).

The addition of nucleotides to Similac Advance infant formula has not been found to boost the immunity of bottle-fed infants in the way that breast milk does for breastfed babies. All the same, this does not deter the manufacturer from creating an advertisement that contains the dubious highlighted statement quoted above. Evidently, the infant formula industry can create without impunity advertisements that boast imaginary benefits of infant formula.

The culture of bottle-feeding has become so deeply ingrained in the American psyche that infant feeding is no longer a matter of providing nourishment for the optimal health and well-being of infants and children. Rather, it has become a cultural phenomenon that reflects parents' views on parenting, women's perspectives on mothering and mother-infant bonding, and parents' visions of family life. In a sense this has all come about because the infant formula industry has used savvy advertising to create a harmful but alluring understanding of infant feeding: infant feeding is no longer about a baby's well-being but more about the baby's parents and their lifestyle.

Over the past century, the infant formula industry has become immensely profitable through the use of effective advertising strategies. In order to keep expanding its consumer base and its profits, the infant formula industry stresses repeatedly in its advertisements the need for women to assert independence from their needy newborns. By not breastfeeding, a woman apparently can and should leave her baby and be comforted greatly by the knowledge that the baby can be nourished with infant formula. The subliminal message that women receive from the onslaught of infant formula advertisements is that mothers should not be bound to babies who need to breastfeed constantly.

4

BREASTFEEDING

BREAST MILK

About nine years ago, I read a *Los Angeles* magazine article in which a popular actress expresses amazement that she can extract so much milk from her breasts. She had discovered the potent nature of breastfeeding, as if by serendipity, even though the majority of women throughout history have appreciated the wonders of breastfeeding. In the modern era, there are numerous countries all over the world that embrace breastfeeding. It is only in the developed world, however, that many women need to learn on their own about the power and benefits of breastfeeding.

I personally could not have imagined how much breast milk I would produce while my son was hospitalized after his preterm birth. He was first fed breast milk through a thin plastic tube that was inserted down his throat and pushed through his esophagus into his stomach. It was terrible to see him gagging on the tube, but the purpose of tube feeding was to enable him to expend as much energy as possible toward growing. Later, it was both relieving and exciting to see him graduate to bottle-feedings of breast milk. Throughout his hospitalization, the primary and consistent way in which I could demonstrate my devotion was to visit him frequently and offer him pumped breast milk.

I was not alone in feeling that I was doing something valuable for my son by expressing breast milk. One evening, as I sat by my son's isolette in the nursery, I overheard the nurse who had treated my son less than gently in the first hours of his life. She was speaking over the telephone to the mother of one of the other babies. The nursery had run out of breast milk for the woman's baby, and the nurse wanted permission to use infant formula. The nurse was unhappy after she hung up the telephone, and she accused the mother aloud of wanting "to starve the baby."

Within twenty minutes, the mother rushed into the nursery with bags of breast milk and complained justly that she had not been told her supply of breast milk had run low. She wanted her baby to have the breast milk that she worked hard to produce for his sake. As I listened, I understood exactly how this mother felt. However sincere the mother was, the nurse remained indignant. Like many health practitioners, the nurse probably did not know much about either breastfeeding or breast milk.

During my medical training in the 1980s, I learned little about breast milk. In my senior year of medical school, I prepared a short presentation on the topic of human milk versus infant formula feeding for preterm infants. I did a great deal of research and tried to evaluate the differences between the two modes of infant feeding. I focused only on the major nutrients contained in both human milk and infant formula and was oblivious to the many other ingredients that human milk alone contained. Thus, I was at a loss to answer my professor when she asked me which of the two modes of infant feeding would be better for a preterm infant. From a superficial analysis of the major nutritional components, the data made it appear as if infant formula was not much different from breast milk.

After my son's preterm birth only a few years later, however, I knew differently. I would have told my professor unequivocally that breast milk is far superior to infant formula. For example, the colostrum of mothers of preterm babies is three times as potent as the colostrum of mothers of term babies (Montagu 1986, 75). Colostrum is a powerful laxative that expels sticky meconium from the infant's gut. It also contains a rich complement of immunoglobulins and protective factors that provide the baby with immunity, including significant protection from diarrhea.

In medical school, however, I learned little about colostrum and breast milk since I was hardly exposed to breastfeeding. Nearly all hospitalized infants, including preterm infants in the Neonatal Intensive Care Unit, were fed infant formula. In fact, a great deal of the nursing work in pediatrics revolves around feeding babies infant formula. Whereas my pediatric training contained practically no education about breastfeeding whatsoever, I was exposed constantly to infant formula products and their sales representatives.

For instance, wherever and whenever pediatricians gathered in medical school or during pediatric residency for conferences, lectures, and group lunches, the infant formula representatives or their company's freebies were omnipresent. Free snacks and meals were often sponsored by infant formula companies. Meanwhile, infant formula logos were imprinted on diverse items (including notepads, paper for daily progress notes, pens, pencils, emergency cards, prescription pads, journals, and books) that were presented for free to students and doctors. Throughout my training, the use of infant formula was treated as an indispensable part of pediatric practice.

NATURALLY SWEET BREAST MILK

When I was in private practice, an infant formula representative once did the crudest of experiments in our office lab. He filled three small paper cups with different infant formulas and asked me to decide which tasted the best. Obliging him, I tasted the samples and assessed his company's to be the most palatable of the three.

Prior to this impromptu taste test, I was unaware that his company's infant formula was sweetened with sucrose, commonly known as table sugar. Sucrose is composed of two sugars, glucose and fructose. Breast milk and most other infant formulas, on the other hand, owe their sweetness to the sugar lactose.

Lactose is found only in mother's milk, including human beings and cows; it is not found in plants. Breast milk, unlike infant formulas, contains the enzyme lactase which metabolizes lactose into glucose and galactose. Lactose has been found to enhance calcium absorption, possibly prevent the development of rickets (Vitamin D deficiency), and provide a readily available source of galactose which is used to produce galactolipids that are essential to brain development (Lawrence 1995, 125). Lactose also provides an instant supply of glucose, which is critical to infant development since glucose is the human brain's only source of energy.

Recent research demonstrates that the brain's reserve of glucose is depleted quickly when human beings face significant cognitive challenges (Murray 2000). Behavioral researchers at the University of Virginia found that glucose improves human memory and attention. In one experiment, elderly people were given lemonade that was sweetened with glucose or saccharin prior to taking tests that measured their short-term memory, attention, and motor function. Those who had drunk glucose-sweetened lemonade recalled nearly twice as much narrative prose as their counterparts who had drunk saccharin-sweetened lemonade.

Analogously, one can surmise the importance of supplying infants with a ready supply of glucose. Infants experience significant amounts of learning as their brains more than double in size during the first year of life. Healthy infants should receive adequate supplies of glucose and galactose in their diet, which can be achieved best by breastfeeding. Moreover, the combination of a readily available source of glucose in lactose and frequent feedings may permit breastfed babies to replenish their stores of glucose in their brains often.

BREAST IS BEST

Hundreds of scientific studies have been done over the past few decades, and they document the unsurpassable benefits of breast milk. Breastfed babies experience a lower incidence of numerous ailments and illnesses, and they have also been shown to score higher on intelligence tests. Although the superiority of breast milk has been established definitively, one would hardly know this in light of the small percentage of women who exclusively breastfeed their babies.

In an effort to encourage more women to breastfeed, overwhelming emphasis is placed upon the importance of breast milk. More women are beginning to see the value of breastfeeding because science continues to elucidate the unique nature of breast milk. In a way, the current trend is the opposite of what occurred in infant feeding a century ago. At the turn of the twentieth century, women became beholden to the science of infant feeding and the use of artificial milk substitutes since physicians had access to scientific information that was not available to the general public.

Historian Rima D. Apple (1987, 27) describes in *Mothers and Medicine: A Social History of Infant Feeding 1890–1950* how physicians meticulously formulated recipes for human milk substitutes. Physicians calculated percentages of fat and sugar and changed the prescriptions constantly. At one point, the pediatrician Luther Emmett Holt prescribed nineteen different formulas for babies in the first year of life alone. Although infant feeding had always been straightforward since the majority of women breastfed, it increasingly became a complex and confusing subject that needed clarification by experts. In the quest to provide their infants with optimal nourishment, women became highly dependent upon physicians and their various infant formulas.

A century later, it has become patently clear from many scientific studies that human milk is irreproducible and far superior to any substitute. As the benefits of breastfeeding continue to be better publicized, more parents are beginning to appreciate the advantages of providing their babies with breast milk. Parents may choose to breastfeed for different reasons, like the obvious benefits of increasing babies' immunity to illnesses and possibly boosting their children's IQ scores. As invaluable as these benefits are, however, the value of breastfeeding itself should not be diminished by overemphasizing the tangible benefits of breastfeeding. There is much more to breastfeeding than the provision of mother's milk.

Consider the following observation made by journalist Lillian Ross (1997, 27) when she interviewed post-partum mothers who were exercising vigorously in Central Park. In the *New Yorker* magazine, Ross describes the mother of a crying ten-week-old baby: "His mom, one of the lawyers, picks him up, pulls out a businesslike breast, firmly sticks the baby's face on it, and says, 'I'm getting, like, more and more O.K. about going back to work.'" This mother approaches breastfeeding with little detectable warmth, and the depiction of this mother-infant breastfeeding dyad is telling: it is a classic example of how one can intellectually comprehend the value of breast milk without actually appreciating the art of breastfeeding. There is far more to breastfeeding than the mere production of breast milk, no matter how powerful and wondrous its components may be.

BREASTFEEDING THE NEWBORN

Breastfeeding is much more than a mere source of oral nourishment. The simple activity of breastfeeding relays to a newborn that he is loved, important, worthy, and an integral part of his family, a group of people that cares deeply about his well-being. Breastfeeding is an intimate and loving display of human affection that every baby deserves to receive since it encourages optimal growth and development.

Although most healthy babies will learn how to breastfeed if they are given the opportunity, the absence of a mother's breast immediately after birth is often a significant impediment to successful breastfeeding. As mentioned earlier, hospital personnel do not hesitate to separate the mother-newborn dyad; sometimes hours may pass before a mother embraces her newborn. Far from being benign, prolonged separation may interfere with the newborn's ability to learn how to breastfeed.

Neonatologist Marshall Klaus and his colleagues (1995, 63) espouse the importance of bonding between mother and newborn as soon as possible after birth. Swedish investigators studied healthy newborns that were dried and placed upon their mothers' abdomens soon after birth. A specific sequence of events occurs as the newborn lies on his mother, warmed by her body heat and a towel. After thirty minutes of resting and occasionally looking up at his mother, the newborn invariably moves upward by pushing with his legs. Most likely guided by the scent of his mother's breast, the newborn finds the areola and begins to suckle without assistance. This sequence of events has been photographed and is well documented.

Ideally, a newborn should learn to breastfeed within minutes of his birth. Given the opportunity to breastfeed early in life, every healthy infant can learn to breastfeed from his mother. This will benefit his mother's uterus, and it will also stimulate the newborn's immature digestive tract to function as it did not have to in the womb. Breastfeeding may be natural behavior, but it must be learned just as everything else in human behavior is learned. This means that a baby needs to be exposed to the breast in order to learn the art of breastfeeding.

My son ultimately received the benefit of nearly three years of breastfeeding, but what was remarkable was that he did not nurse at the breast until he was five weeks old. My first attempt to nurse him at the breast was inept, and I felt as if I was offering his small mouth a mountain of a breast. Fortunately, I had the assistance of a wonderful nurse who suggested a few tips on getting my son to latch on to the breast. It took him a few trials, but he learned quickly.

I was also fortunate that my daughter learned to breastfeed because I was not well toward the end of my second pregnancy. I developed massive fluid retention and high blood pressure after being placed on bed rest and a medication to prevent preterm labor. After I gave birth, the maternity nurse insisted that I be concerned with my own health instead of worrying about breastfeeding my daughter. I could hardly argue since I had two IVs, a painful urinary catheter, and significant edema throughout my entire body. I was fortunate, however, that the separation from my newborn did not impair irreparably my ability to breastfeed her.

Since the majority of women experience childbirth in hospitals, many women face the probability of being separated from their newborns. With more than one-fourth of babies being born by cesarean section, it is unsurprising that breastfeeding often becomes a secondary issue of concern. After such a disruptive experience, the well-being of the mother is nearly always a matter that is considered separately from the well-being of the newborn. Additionally, a mother is often permitted to hold her baby only briefly since many babies who are born via cesarean section have health problems that need to be addressed not in their mothers' arms but in the nursery. The separation of the mother-newborn dyad may occur for what appears to be sound reasons, but the disruption of the mother-newborn bond can have long-lasting effects.

I know several women who wound up unable to breastfeed their newborns after undergoing cesarean births. One friend had difficulty bonding with her newborn, and her troubles were compounded by her inability to produce sufficient breast milk. Intervention with a lactation consultant was only moderately helpful. My friend did not breastfeed beyond a few weeks, and she confided that her baby seemed much more comfortable with his grandmother.

I have also heard of women who wanted to breastfeed but were not taught how or why they needed to pump their breasts. For instance, my sister told me of two friends who were separated from their newborns because one was born preterm. and the other was ill. Neither woman received assistance in learning how to pump her breasts. Subsequently, each woman experienced great difficulty with breastfeeding.

Simply stated, there are many women who are not given proper instructions about breastfeeding either before or after giving birth. Since breastfeeding is most definitely a learned ability, hospitals must provide new mothers with proper education regarding the techniques of breastfeeding and breast pumping. Proper breastfeeding education is being introduced in some hospitals, particularly by those that are certified to promote breastfeeding by Baby Friendly, USA under the auspices of United Children's Fund (UNICEF) and the World Health Organization (WHO).

As a new mother, I was lucky that my son was born in a hospital that provided sufficient support for breastfeeding mothers. Once the choice of breastfeeding was recorded on my medical chart, the maternity nurses followed their protocol of helping me to learn how to use a breast pump. Initially, breastfeeding might have been a choice of infant feeding, but it eventually became an indispensable resource for nurturing the healthy growth and development of both my children.

SUCKLING AT THE BREAST

My son was hospitalized for forty days, and I seemed to have developed an ostensibly closer relationship to my rented electric breast pump than I did to my baby. At the time he began to breastfeed, I was delighted that he was nursing, and I quickly forgot that he might not have learned how to suckle at the breast. It turned out that we were fortunate since some babies do not succeed in learning how to suckle at the breast.

Although sucking and suckling are assumed to be interchangeable physical acts, they are not. In fact, a baby may get confused if he is offered the breast to suckle for one feeding and then given a bottle to suck on at the next feeding. Ashley Montagu describes the mechanism behind suckling clearly in several of his writings about breastfeeding. (Please see Appendix B for a detailed description of suckling.)

During suckling, the baby's gums and lips press against the areola, which is the pigmented skin around the nipple. The collecting sinuses are located under the areola. As the baby nurses, he establishes a rhythm of suckling, swallowing, and breathing. With proper suckling, the 15–30 pores in the nipple will spurt out fine streams of milk in different directions.

Ashley Montagu (1986, 82) explains that a baby does not suck at the breast since sucking produces a partial vacuum in the baby's mouth, which will invariably cause trauma to his mother's nipple. Sucking, however, is what a baby needs to do to extract liquid from a bottle. If the formula flows too freely through the nipple hole, a baby may need to either thrust his tongue against the nipple or bite down on the nipple to stop the flow of milk. Hence, babies may become confused if they are drinking from both the breast and the bottle.

Improper suckling of the breast may traumatize the nipple and cause enough discomfort to discourage a mother from continuing to breastfeed. Women who wish to breastfeed successfully should try to avoid bottle-feedings in order to prevent nipple confusion. Ideally, the baby should be permitted to suckle at the breast since suckling at the breast affects the baby's physical development.

For instance, suckling requires the concerted action of numerous structures within the mouth and back of the throat, as well as facial structures and muscles. Breastfeeding, by stimulating these various structures and muscles, affects significantly the later development of facial shape, teeth position, and speech. A recent study showed that breastfeeding offers a protective effect against misalignment of primary teeth even when babies used pacifiers or sucked their thumbs (Viggiano et al. 2004). Overall, breastfed babies have a lower incidence of malocclusion, which is the irregular positioning of opposing teeth, such as an overbite or underbite; they also experience fewer speech impediments, including speech delay (Montagu 1986, 86).

LEARNING TO BREASTFEED

Women may be endowed with mammary glands, but they need to learn how to breastfeed since they are not born with an instinct to breastfeed. If women did possess such an instinct, all women would be programmed to automatically and capably breastfeed their newborn babies. Obviously, this is not the case since so many women choose not to breastfeed, and many women find breastfeeding to be challenging.

Biology alone cannot and does not dictate whether or not a woman will choose to breastfeed or if she can succeed with breastfeeding. What is of great significance is what parents have learned from the culture in which they have been reared and what they continue to learn from current cultural influences. Indeed, cultural influences can be so powerful that some childbearing women may never be exposed to breastfeeding.

Culture is what Ashley Montagu (1971) defines as being the "man-made part of the environment, the learned part of the environment." Early in the course of evolution, human beings lost instincts because "predetermined modes of behavior acted as so many impediments" (1971). Since an instinct is a fixed reaction to a given stimulus, human beings would have been stymied if they reacted automatically and unthinkingly to different and difficult challenges presented by an ever-changing environment.

In order for human beings to survive, a high premium was placed upon the ability to think and solve problems. By using the ability to think, human beings were able to create culture. It is through culture that human beings share with one another thought processes, words, and actions; modes of communication; ways to solve problems; the tools and objects that facilitate existence; and anything else that expresses the human abilities to think and act.

Arguably, modern culture does not provide the general public with sufficiently helpful or accurate information about breastfeeding. For example, in the introduction to *A History of the Breast*, historian Marilyn Yalom (1997, 3) asks the following question: "Who owns the breast? Does it belong to the suckling child, whose life is dependent on a mother's milk or an effective substitute?" Although this query might seem valid and straightforward, it is truly unclear in what ways a child's life is actually dependent upon mother's milk.

Breastfeeding was absolutely essential to human survival throughout human existence. It may be true that a mother's breast is no longer the uniquely powerful source of milk that once determined whether or not a baby would survive infancy. The advent of milk pasteurization in the latter half of the nineteenth century improved significantly the sterility of animal milk used to feed young babies. However important this scientific advancement in germ control may have been, the saddest consequence of creating a supposedly safe alternative to breastfeeding has been to diminish the significance of breastfeeding's numerous other benefits.

Although many parents appreciate the concept of high quality in nearly every aspect of child-rearing, the vitally important task of infant nurturing is inexplicably treated almost cavalierly. According to current statistics, the majority of newborns are breastfed but not for long. Since infants consume breast milk or infant formula for the entire first year of life, the majority of American infants are bottle-fed with infant formula. Sadly, even breastfed babies are often given a combination of breast milk and infant formula. In other words, the much touted phrase "breast is best" carries little weight and bears insignificant influence on parents' decision when it comes to infant feeding.

The prevalent perception of breastfeeding is that it is merely an optional mode of infant feeding, one that can be tried but that does not need to be pursued beyond the newborn period. This view of breastfeeding parallels many Americans' understanding of exercise. Although most people are aware that exercise is good for their health and well-being, many do not exercise simply because they either do not wish to or they do not appreciate the need to do so.

In 1999–2000, according to the Centers for Disease Control and Prevention (CDC), 30 percent of American adults were obese and 64 percent were either overweight or obese (Centers for Disease Control 2004c). In the majority of cases, obesity is related to a sedentary lifestyle and excessive food intake that is not balanced with sufficient amounts of exercise or physical exertion. Exercise, like breastfeeding, is highly beneficial for the maintenance of good health and well-being, but both activities are thought to be unnecessary, too difficult, or too cumbersome.

For the longest part of human history, exercise was not an option but a natural part of daily life that kept in equilibrium the intake of nourishment and the expenditure of energy. Similarly, breastfeeding was a definitive way of nourishing babies and bonding with them. Human beings did not have the choice of not exercising or not breastfeeding: they exercised, and women breastfed because both activities were a natural part of daily life. In stark contrast, the once normal, highly productive, and beneficial activities of breastfeeding and exercise are now thought to be optional or even obsolete. In the modern era, it is often by chance that one may understand or learn about the benefits of breastfeeding and exercise.

BREASTFEEDING FOR MOTHER'S HEALTH

As long as breastfeeding is viewed as an optional mode of infant feeding, a skewed view of women's health will persist. The fact is that childbearing women have a biological need to breastfeed. Breastfeeding is highly beneficial for a nursing baby, and it also benefits his mother greatly.

In the newborn period, the hormone oxytocin is released during breastfeeding. Oxytocin plays an important role in normalizing a woman's uterus, which is significant since this unique organ grows and stretches in order to accommodate the presence of a fetus during pregnancy. The uterus needs to return to its normal size after childbirth. Under the influence of oxytocin, numerous blood vessels and muscles in the uterus contract to minimize the bleeding of the womb that occurs after giving birth. Continued breastfeeding helps the uterus contract back to its pre-pregnancy size more quickly. Any woman who has breastfed her newborn knows how powerfully and effectively oxytocin contracts the uterus.

A mother receives many benefits from breastfeeding, including the following (American Academy of Pediatrics 2005):

- decreased bleeding after childbirth;
- uterus normalizes more quickly;
- decreased menstrual blood loss;
- increased spacing between pregnancies;
- quicker return to pre-pregnancy weight;
- decreased risk of breast cancer;
- decreased risk of ovarian cancer;
- possible decreased risk of osteoporosis and hip fractures.

In other words, breastfeeding reduces significantly a mother's loss of blood, provides contraception (that should be supplemented with another form of contraception, like a prophylactic), increases the spacing between pregnancies, decreases the risk of cancer, burns extra calories, and perhaps leads to the maintenance of women's bone strength long after breastfeeding ceases.

Breastfeeding also bestows a calming effect that is produced most probably by the hormone oxytocin in the presence of estrogen (Dermer and Montgomery 1997). There are also studies that demonstrate other benefits of breastfeeding. For example, the longer a woman breastfeeds, the lower her risk is of contracting Rheumatoid Arthritis, which is a chronic and debilitating illness (Karlson et al. 2004). Overall, breastfeeding provides infants and their mothers with immense short-term and long-term emotional, psychological, and biological benefits.

In contrast, fathers do not have a physiological need to breastfeed. In light of the numerous benefits breastfeeding provides both mothers and babies, fathers should support breastfeeding. In fact, the importance of a father's support of breastfeeding was evident in a recent study published in *The American Journal of Obstetrics and Gynecology*.

The study showed that if prospective fathers attended one class on infant care that advocates breastfeeding, 74 percent of their wives breastfed as compared to only 41 percent of women whose spouses attended a class that gave no information on breastfeeding (French 2005). Evidently, fathers play an irreplaceable role in supporting the mutually beneficial relationship of breastfeeding between both mother and infant. Sadly, some fathers may feel slighted or discouraged that their role in early infant care appears to be secondary. Fathers should, however, feel confident that their supportive role early on helps to foster a primary role for both mothers and fathers throughout their children's lives.

DISREGARD FOR BREASTFEEDING

In order for women to lead a life that modern culture will respect, breastfeeding usually does not play a significant role. Women are often expected to disregard their babies' need for intimate maternal care, which includes breastfeeding. It is doubtful, though, that women become mothers in order to learn how to suppress maternal behavior. For the greater part of human existence, women could easily express maternal affection since they were intimately bound to their babies.

Breastfeeding mothers generally stay close to their babies, but such closeness may be regarded with suspicion in the modern era. Women may be criticized for becoming too attached to their babies, or they may be assessed to be neurotic, overprotective, silly, dumb, unreasonable, weird, controlling, overly attached, or living vicariously through their children. Apparently, as wonderful as it is for women to become mothers, they are expected to center their lives upon many relationships and activities that are unrelated to their babies and children.

It hardly seems to matter that doing the work of caring for one's children and home requires a tremendous amount of energy, dedication, and perseverance. Children do not become productive and contributive citizens without being exposed consistently to the environmental stimulation that nurtures such development from early infancy. Homes do not remain clean and comfortable without the time-consuming efforts made mostly by women to maintain their homes.

Women who stay home do a great deal of work, but such work does not generate income.

It is a sad testament to modern society that women who stay home may feel demoralized because they are ostensibly unproductive. Stay-at-home mothers, however, do a great deal of domestic work: they simply do not receive enough respect or admiration for doing such work. As a result, some women may become discouraged by their supposed lack of productivity. Hence, I have heard some stay-at-home mothers say, "I'm only my kids' chauffeur, and I don't do anything...I just take care of my kids."

Of all the work a mother does in the home, the work of breastfeeding is the least appreciated as being bona fide work. Housekeeping is work that includes cooking, grocery shopping, cleaning, doing laundry, vacuuming, tidying, and keeping one's home in good condition. For many women, homemaking also includes management of household finances. The work of caring for babies consists of feeding them, changing their diapers and clothing, cleaning them, as well as playing and interacting with them. These activities are not abstract, and they need to be performed to maintain the stability of one's home and the health of one's baby. The current perception of breastfeeding, on the other hand, is that it is an expendable activity that is of dubious value since the use of infant formula is so common.

MISUNDERSTANDING BREASTFEEDING

The widespread availability of infant formula assures many women that bottle-feeding is a practical and reasonable form of infant feeding. Thus, there will be situations in which women may succeed with breastfeeding yet fail to appreciate its myriad benefits. For instance, a friend of mine had a cesarean section, and she encountered some difficulties with breastfeeding: her breasts were frequently engorged, her son spit up frequently, and he caught colds. She did not enjoy her breastfeeding experience, so she stopped after six months: she was not at all convinced that breastfeeding had benefited her son. After she gave birth to her second child via an elective cesarean section, she did not even bother to breastfeed.

My friend might not have appreciated breastfeeding, but her perspective was based upon a limited understanding of breastfeeding. When one assumes that breastfeeding will be an easy and uneventful experience because it is natural, one mistakenly forgets about all the medical interference that impairs the breastfeeding relationship in the first place. Before denouncing breastfeeding, it would be more worthwhile to examine thoroughly which factors are responsible for triggering the dysfunctional breastfeeding relationship. One cannot isolate breastfeeding as an activity that exists independently of other life circumstances.

Indeed, the prolonged physical separation of a newborn from her mother has been shown to affect maternal behavior negatively. If a mother is separated from her baby for too long, she might not become as absorbed in her baby's well-being. Cesarean births complicate matters greatly for the breastfeeding dyad since mothers are often separated from their newborns for hours, and many mothers experience discomfort from the surgery. The wound takes time to heal, and it may be difficult for women to breastfeed comfortably: it is physically challenging for women to breastfeed their newborns every hour or two after having undergone major abdominal surgery.

In contrast, babies in some hunter-gatherer cultures nurse as frequently as every ten to fifteen minutes around the clock. In such cultures, the baby is born naturally and without anesthesia, nearly always carried during the day by the mother, and kept snuggled next to her breastfeeding mother at nighttime. Such breastfeeding practices have helped women nurture their children throughout human history, but they are not readily understood any longer.

For instance, during my pediatric residency, I met a woman who was exasperated by her baby's frequent crying. She wound up paying a pediatric gastroenterologist $350 for an hour-long consultation to learn that her healthy four-month-old baby was hungry. The baby could not comply with her mother's scheduled feedings of every three to four hours. Although the mother understood the benefits of breastfeeding, she had difficulty comprehending the flexibility she needed to satisfy her nursling's hunger.

In the bottle-feeding era, it has become customary to feed babies every three to four hours on regimented schedules. This type of feeding schedule arose primarily because it takes that long for infant formula to be digested. Breastfed babies, however, need to nurse more frequently than every three to four hours since breast milk is easily digestible. Unfortunately, parents may expect their babies to breastfeed less often, and they may become confounded when their babies cry and need to nurse frequently at the breast.

With better education and more support for breastfeeding, it is possible to view breastfeeding as a simple and natural part of daily life, much as hunter-gatherers perceived it to be. Child-rearing practices that accommodate breastfeeding can certainly be adapted to modern-day living in the Western World. For now, the prevailing mind-set about breastfeeding is that it is difficult.

DIFFICULTIES WITH BREASTFEEDING

While it is true that some women are able to breastfeed easily and seemingly naturally, other women find breastfeeding to be difficult. The majority of mothers and their babies need both time and first-hand experience before they feel fully at ease with breastfeeding and appreciate its many benefits and convenience. Again, because there is no instinct that drives women to breastfeed, the activity of breastfeeding must be treated as a learning endeavor.

As with all else in life, learning encompasses trial and error, as well as confusion and possible failure. With perseverance and dedication, however, most women will be able to breastfeed successfully. The general consensus appears to be that by six weeks the majority of nursing mothers will have become comfortable with breastfeeding. Even so, there may be situations in which women will not be able to breastfeed.

For example, I have a friend whose baby could not latch on to the breast properly even after lengthy visits with a lactation consultant. Understanding and respecting the benefits of breastfeeding, my friend chose to pump her breasts for ten months so that her daughter could receive expressed breast milk. She looked for a different solution after she realized that it would be fairly impossible to nurture her daughter at the breast. Pumping her breasts required consistent dedication and work, but she was willing to do this for her daughter.

There will be other situations when fortitude and patience will enable a woman to succeed with breastfeeding. My sister, for instance, gave birth to a healthy baby boy in 2001 and experienced great difficulty with breastfeeding from the outset. The baby nursed well, but my sister experienced pain whenever he breastfed. Despite the discomfort, my sister persisted with breastfeeding. After a couple of weeks, the problem was diagnosed: my sister was found to have a serious and widespread Candida yeast infection that afflicted both her breasts.

In general, the growth of yeast is normally checked by bacteria, but this balance can be upset in the presence of antibiotics. My sister had received antibiotics prophylactically during childbirth. Since both of her nipples had become infected with Candida, they were severely cracked and tender to touch. As a result, my sister experienced excruciating discomfort whenever her baby suckled, which was frequently.

My sister suffered for months before she could eradicate the infection. Complicating matters further, she had an active let down that resulted in her breasts leaking milk constantly. Despite the terrible pain and the inconvenience breastfeeding appeared to create, however, my sister persevered with breastfeeding because she understood its long-term benefits. Although breastfeeding was problematic early on, the convenience and benefits she experienced subsequently were priceless.

5

IN SUPPORT OF BREASTFEEDING

A SUPPORTIVE BREASTFEEDING ENVIRONMENT

My sister was fortunate since she had her husband's encouragement to breastfeed their younger son. For many months my sister undertook breastfeeding as a full-time job. She walked bare-chested in her home so that she could air dry the delicate skin of her traumatized and infected breasts. Her husband supported her as she suffered through her difficulties and helped her to persevere with breastfeeding.

For many families today, even as homes have become more stylish and better equipped with amenities, it is not a simple matter to create a warm environment that encourages breastfeeding. The primary goal of most families today has little to do with permitting a mother to stay home and breastfeed her newborn infant. Instead, it is argued that women no longer need to stay home with young children, especially when financial obligations force them to work outside the home.

In order to live a comfortable middle-class lifestyle today, more and more women work outside the home and leave the care of their young babies and children to others. For the many women who return to work outside the home, breastfeeding is a low priority since they are preoccupied with many other concerns. Even though they may have recently experienced the life-altering experience of giving birth, they need to organize baby care placement and anticipate the stress of returning to work outside the home after taking fairly short maternity leaves.

According to the International Labour Organization (ILO), "The maternity and nursing benefits given to working mothers in the United States are the least generous in the industrialized world" (Atkinson 2003). In a February 16, 1998, *Washington Post* article entitled "Study: U.S. Mothers Face Stingy Maternity Benefits; U.N. Agency Finds Disparity With Other Nations," Kirstin Downey Grimsley notes the following: "The report, which reviewed maternity leave and health benefits mandated by law in 152 countries, found that about 80 percent of countries offer paid maternity leave to women workers; about a third of the countries permit the leaves to last for more than 14 weeks." F.J. Dy-Hammer, chief of ILO's work-conditions department, who oversaw the study offers the following observation: "My colleagues and I say that in the United States, it's a do-it-yourself maternity plan." The United States grants new mothers only the Family and Medical Leave Act, which was passed in 1993 and allows employees to take up to 12 weeks of unpaid leave for medical reasons, including childbirth.

Complicating matters further for women who return to work outside the home is the harsh reality that the majority will probably earn and take home less income than their husbands. In an April 7, 1997, *USA Today* article entitled "Tax Laws no Friend of Working Mothers," Edward McCaffery writes that tax specialists found that a woman who works outside the home for an income of $40,000 per year could wind up with $1,000 in real earnings. Taxes account for the vast reduction in net income since they may add up to 50 percent of a mother's salary.

McCaffery also cites the "non-tax costs of holding down a job: child-care expenses, commuting, dry cleaning, clothing, housekeeping, restaurant meals, and time-saving but more expensive in-home food. All these additional non-tax costs might add up to $20,000 a year—offset only by a $1,000 or less child-care tax credit." Consequently, even as many women with young children may return to work outside the home in order to pay bills, they might not be well compensated for their efforts and sacrifices. Additionally, it is difficult to measure the indeterminate price tag of a baby's well-being.

PUTTING BABY AND BREASTFEEDING FIRST

Ideally, every baby should have a loving mother who is willing and available to breastfeed on demand. This makes sense since human beings are mammals, and mammals nurse their babies. When breastfeeding becomes a way of life, parents place a baby's well-being first and foremost; recognize the needs of a baby; comprehend the long-term benefits of better physical, mental, and psychological health for both mother and baby; and understand the importance of a mother's presence in her baby's life. If parents view breastfeeding as a way of life, they can see that breastfeeding on demand is a full-time job that encourages the healthy development of not only a child's life but her parents' lives as well.

Parents who choose to put the well-being of young children first will reap the benefits of their children's healthy growth and development. After all, parents live together with their children, and it is impossible to separate the well-being of children from that of their parents. In fact, breastfeeding assures parents that they do not separate themselves from their young children, particularly when the latter are immature and need the love and nurturing of caring adults.

Breastfeeding is an all-encompassing source of life nourishment, an activity that expresses unequivocally a mother's unconditional love. It is this unconditional love that young babies (and human beings at any age) need so profoundly. Many adults, however, misunderstand the human need for unconditional love.

I am a person who long misunderstood the word *love*, and I do not recall encountering the term *unconditional love* until after I had my children. My father was often cruel, insensitive, and he had difficulty expressing his love until he approached the end of his life. By then my mother could hardly forgive him for the pain he had caused her, but my sister and I were able to forge new bonds with him. My sister is a most loving and generous human being, so I simply followed her example of loving our father. It was a timely renewal of our relationship since he passed away only a year later.

Love is a difficult concept to comprehend, but Ashley Montagu offers an insightful and meaningful description (1970, 466–467):

1. Love is not only a subjective feeling which one has, an emotion, but a series of acts by means of which one conveys to another the feeling that one is deeply involved, profoundly interested, in them and in their welfare. In this sense love is demonstrative, it is sacrificial, it is self-abnegative. It puts the other always first. It is not a cold or calculated altruism, but a deep complete involvement with another.

2. Love is unconditional, it makes no bargains, it trades with no one for anything. It conveys the feeling, the in-the-bone belief, that you are all for the other, that you are always available to give him your support, to contribute to his development as best you can. Love values the other for what he is, not because he is something you want or expect him to be.

3. Love is supportive; it conveys to the other that you will never commit the supreme treason that one human being can commit against another, namely, failure or desertion when you are most needed. Love promises

> that you will always be present to support the other and that no matter what the conditions you will never fail to offer yourself; that you will neither condemn, nor condone, but that you will always be there to offer your sympathy and your understanding; and that whatever the other needs as a human being he shall have, even though it may be a firm "No." Love means that you will be there to help him say "Yes" to life, and to help him have his needs for love satisfied.

After reading this profound definition of love, it occurred to me how easily breastfeeding allowed me to express my love for my children. By letting the children nurse at the breast consistently, I showed them that I was there for them. The intimate contact of breastfeeding transmitted to them my love for them. Regardless of my mood, the breasts were there to provide my children dependable nourishment, unconditional love, and intimate human contact.

There is little doubt that a mother can use breastfeeding to provide her child love, irrespective of how unaffectionate she might actually feel when the child happens to need it. As adults, it is not always easy to express love consistently to young children. This is because human beings experience the fluctuations of constantly changing moods that occur in response to varying circumstances in daily life.

Although some parents weather the vicissitudes of life well, others do not. As a parent who could not always remain calm and collected, I hoped to extend to my children the consistency of something deeper and unchanging—my love. Breastfeeding was the resource I used to convey unfailing love for my children in spite of my occasional moodiness.

THE DISRUPTED ART OF BREASTFEEDING

Historian Rima D. Apple describes in *Mothers and Medicine* how physicians attributed high infant mortality and morbidity to improper infant feeding in the second half of the nineteenth century. In the 1860s a German chemist named Justus von Liebig was concerned about the health of infants who were not breastfed. According to Apple (1987, 6), he formulated a mixture of fats, carbohydrates, and proteins that would provide the basic nutritive elements of human milk; his product was marketed in the United States in 1869. Meanwhile, other chemists like Henri Nestlé were creating their own infant food products.

The new infant food industry detected the large potential demand for its products, and it colluded with the medical establishment to wrest control of infant feeding from mothers. The industry created advertisements that boasted the wonders of artificial milk and referred mothers to the care of physicians who prescribed the infant formulas. Whereas the greater majority of women had nurtured their babies intuitively at the breast throughout history, the infant food industry and physicians informed women that they no longer possessed the knowledge or wisdom to nourish their own babies.

As more women relied on medical expertise to feed their infants, greater dependence upon artificial feeding arose. Physicians used their knowledge of science to quantify calories and percentages of nutrients; they impressed upon mothers the superiority of scientific information over maternal intuition. Motherly wisdom was abandoned wholesale so that women could learn to obey higher authorities, such as physicians.

Apparently, women did not subscribe blindly to the trend toward artificial feeding over breastfeeding. Apple (1987, 19) explains that women were intrigued by the science of infant feeding and wanted the best for their babies:

> In their desire to provide the best care for their children, American mothers relied increasingly on experts. A combination of sophisticated advertising techniques, the aura of scientific motherhood, and the vaunted expertise of the medical profession—an interplay of ideology and material factors—created an atmosphere that motivated many women to seek out commercial products and medical advice. The commercialization and medicalization of infant care established an environment that made artificial feeding not only acceptable to many mothers but also "natural" and "necessary."

It is unclear, however, if women understood the enormity of what they gave up when they ceded their autonomy as thinking mothers in order to become listening and obeying mothers.

At the same time that breastfeeding was being overtaken by the burgeoning use of artificial feeding, home childbirth in the care of midwives was shifting toward hospitalized childbirth under the care of physicians who administered anesthesia and used invasive procedures. The practices of both childbirth and infant feeding would be changed indelibly for decades to come.

In truth, it is inconceivable that medical practitioners would have advocated the use of infant formula at the turn of the twentieth century. Refrigeration and water sanitation then were not at all what it is today. Living conditions a century ago were abominable for many people, particularly immigrants in urban areas. Many families were squeezed into crowded and unsanitary tenements.

In her memoir, physician S. Josephine Baker (1992, 153–154) describes the terrible living conditions faced by countless poor New Yorkers in 1902:

> In my district, the heart of old Hell's Kitchen on the west side, the heat, the smells, the squalor made it something not to be believed.... I climbed stair after stair, knocked on door after door, met drunk after drunk, filthy mother after filthy mother and dying baby after dying baby.... It was an appalling summer too, with an average of fifteen hundred babies dying each week in the city; lean, miserable, wailing little souls carried off wholesale by dysentery.... Babies always died in summer and there was no point in trying to do anything about it.

As a pioneer of the preventive health movement, Dr. Baker did a great deal to prevent infant morbidity and mortality in New York City.

In the summer of 1908, she worked as an executive in the New York City Department of Health and hired nurses to visit mothers and their newborns in "a complicated, filthy, sunless, and stifling nest of tenements on the lower east side of the city" (1992, 156). They would try to determine whether or not preventive health measures could decrease the rate of infant mortality in an era when thousands of babies died from diarrhea during the hottest months of the summer. She directed the nurses, who had been trained in baby care, to visit newborns and their mothers as soon as possible after birth.

The nurses advised mothers with common sense: "Nothing revolutionary; just insistence on breast-feeding, efficient ventilation, frequent bathing, the right kind of thin summer clothes, out-of-door airing in the little strip of park around the corner—all of it common place enough for the modern baby...all of it new in public health" (1992, 156). The results of the experiment were impressive. While the rest of the city experienced terrible infant mortality as usual that summer, Dr. Baker's emphasis on breastfeeding and hygiene decreased the mortality of infants in the experimental district by 1,200.

Dr. Baker's inspiring work in preventive health care demonstrated the importance of breastfeeding and hygiene in reducing infant mortality. Although she might have understood the importance of breastfeeding, she was nevertheless an early supporter of providing babies a more uniform infant formula as opposed to individually prescribed formulas. Dr. Baker helped to establish baby health stations in New York City to provide health care and infant formula to babies (Apple 1987, 76).

UNDERMINING BREASTFEEDING

Historian Rima D. Apple (1987, 127–128) explains that physicians undermined women's confidence in breastfeeding by prescribing measures that made them nearly neurotic. Physicians overemphasized the importance of producing optimally nourishing breast milk and advised some breastfeeding mothers to supplement with feedings of bottled formula. For example, women at Madison General Hospital in Wisconsin were permitted to breastfeed, "but breast-fed infants were weighed before and after each feeding to determine how much bottle formula was needed to supplement the mother's milk supply" (127–128). Apple (128) notes that this protocol was followed in hospitals "despite the recognition that such feeding could decrease the stimulation of the mother's breasts needed to promote maternal nursing."

Physicians also monitored diets, recommended regular exercise, and checked women's temperaments in order to optimize the nourishment offered to breast-fed babies. These exhaustive prescriptive measures did not help many women. Instead, they had the opposite effect of leading women to think that their breast milk was not good enough for their babies. As a result of this medical interference, women's confidence in breastfeeding plummeted, and more women sought recommendations for artificial milk substitutes from their physicians.

Physicians might have professed to improve the quality of breast milk with prescriptive health measures, but they wound up stripping women of motherly intuition and discouraging them from breastfeeding. By the 1950s the art of breastfeeding was nearly eradicated, and physicians recommended only the use of artificial milk. Although the original intention of physicians might have been to provide young babies with optimal nutrition, breastfeeding mothers were actually taught that their breast milk supply was inadequate and insufficiently nourishing.

Breastfeeding may be better understood better now than it was fifty years ago, but many health practitioners still do not have much confidence in breastfeeding. Even those who support breastfeeding may wind up discouraging women from nursing. A prevalent concern health practitioners still have with breastfeeding is that a breastfed baby might not be receiving adequate nourishment.

For instance, my daughter weighed six pounds and three ounces at birth, but she weighed exactly six pounds at her two-week check-up. The nurse practitioner was troubled by my daughter's weight loss even though my breasts were full of milk, and my baby was nursing well and wetting plenty of diapers. I was advised to continue nursing my daughter, but we were to schedule a follow-up weight check two weeks later in the office. At her two-month check-up, my exclusively breastfed daughter doubled her weight to twelve pounds, and she looked like a little rotund cherub.

There is little doubt that my education and experience with babies helped me to gauge accurately the status of my baby's well-being. She was alert, suckling frequently at the breast, well hydrated since her mouth was moist, and soaking her diapers. I was assured of my daughter's well-being, and I knew what to look for in case her health was in any way jeopardized. Understandably, many breastfeeding mothers who have not been trained similarly might lose confidence in their ability to breastfeed exclusively.

I mention this experience to clarify how simple it is to discourage and confuse a breastfeeding mother. As a mother who had already exclusively breastfed one child, I was confident that exclusive breastfeeding was healthy and correct. In contrast, many breastfeeding mothers are cautioned far too frequently that they might not have enough breast milk or that they risk endangering their babies' well-being by not supplementing with infant formula or glucose water.

When more women gain greater experience with breastfeeding, however, other women will also feel more confident about their ability to breastfeed. A healthy mother-infant dyad that remains in close contact will create an abundant supply of breast milk and have no need for artificial supplements. Such confidence is not reflected, unfortunately, in breastfeeding statistics.

The positive news is that the 2003 breastfeeding initiation rate of 62.5 percent in hospitals was close to the goal of 75 percent (Li et al. 2003). The rate of continuation was not as encouraging since it was 27 percent at 6 months and 12.3 percent at 12 months, as compared to the goals of 50 percent at 6 months and 25 percent at 12 months (Li et al. 2003). More women are breastfeeding initially, but the fall off is significant, and the use of infant formula supplements is still common.

In fact, researchers have noted that even though women say they are breastfeeding, many are also using infant formula supplements. Hence, there is often some confusion as to what extent babies are actually being breastfed when researchers study breastfeeding. Suffice it to say that more women are breastfeeding, which is an excellent trend, but the majority of healthy babies continue to be fed infant formula.

BREASTFEEDING ADVOCATES

Over the course of a century, physicians helped to create the bottle-feeding culture that nearly eradicated the art of breastfeeding. Sound education is the only effective way to reverse the unfortunate legacy of a century-long campaign that sought systematically to discourage women from breastfeeding. From this perspective, grassroots educational movements like La Leche League have helped many women benefit from breastfeeding. This organization's most prominent book is aptly entitled *The Womanly Art of Breastfeeding*. Although I did not participate in the league, I was encouraged by two physicians who were active supporters.

These two pediatricians were well known among pediatric residents in Los Angeles as being unequivocal supporters of breastfeeding. When I began working in private practice, one of the pediatricians kindly sent me a box of books and articles about breastfeeding in response to my inquiry about gaining access to good breastfeeding resources. Prior to encountering these physicians, I had thought and learned little about breastfeeding.

Toward the end of my pediatric residency, I met a woman whose adolescent daughter had been cared for by one of these pediatricians for many years. The mother was proud that her daughter had been breastfed for exactly three years. Her pediatrician had recommended this, and she had trusted him enough to follow his advice.

Although women have been taught for the past century that breastfeeding is an inadequate and insufficient source of nourishment for babies, the truth is that breastfeeding is optimal. Babies need to breastfeed. The art of breastfeeding must be learned once again, and future teachers will be mothers who have breastfed so that they can show others how to breastfeed.

Just as I have been encouraged by the breastfeeding mothers I have met, I know that sharing knowledge and wisdom of breastfeeding's wonders will encourage many other women to do the same for their children. Indubitably, the culture of breastfeeding can be created anew so that breastfeeding will again become an integral part of a healthy and wise way of life. The art of breastfeeding needs to be shared not only between a mother and her nursing baby but with the rest of society. Society will become much more humane when breastfeeding babies are part of the normal landscape of American daily life.

6

THE ART OF BREASTFEEDING

BREASTFEEDING AND COMMUNICATION

Parenting may become difficult and unpleasant when parents are unable to communicate with their babies or toddlers. I have witnessed the same scenario too often, one in which a young baby or toddler is screaming at the top of her lungs, and her parents cannot calm her down. Bystanders generally intensify the situation by staring or glaring at the inconsolable child and helpless parents.

The majority of parents are unaware that there is a most efficacious tool available to calm babies and toddlers easily and successfully: it is breastfeeding. Most babies and toddlers are calmed immediately by breastfeeding, and they will express contentment by simply crying less or not at all. In most circumstances, breastfeeding offers a baby or toddler a clear signal that there is comfort and satisfaction ahead. It is terrible at any age to experience dissatisfaction or the travails associated with poor communication.

When faced with a situation in which communication is difficult or impossible, some parents may view a baby's lack of cooperative behavior as a sign of her willful disobedience. This interpretation of a baby's behavior may lead parents to withhold their love and affection or use strategies like time outs or corporal punishment. This is done in an effort to instill discipline, avoid being manipulated, and making sure children know that it is the parents who are in control. Unfortunately, many of these tactics fail to transmit sincere parental concern and love to the distressed children.

Breastfeeding, on the other hand, imparts to young children parental sympathy and understanding as well as an offer of pleasure and satisfaction. Even in the most challenging of circumstances, breastfeeding can provide young children a universal sign of caring communication. Undoubtedly, one of the reasons infants and toddlers need to nurse frequently is simply to interact intimately and frequently with a nurturing caregiver. The more often a baby interacts with her breastfeeding mother, the more often she will be able to learn the art and discipline of living as a human being.

Every time a baby breastfeeds, she learns something at the breast. She will hear her mother say different things, feel the temperature of her mother's skin change as the climate changes, sense different moods her mother experiences, and learn how pleasurable it is to be nourished at the breast. She will also learn how responsive her breastfeeding mother is to her myriad needs. In other words, breastfeeding opens channels of communication.

A parent's ability to comfort a baby is a definitive sign of efficacious communication. By using the tool of breastfeeding, a sleepy and cranky baby can fall back to sleep in almost any location, an ill and uncomfortable baby can be reassured, a frightened baby on an airplane can be soothed by the familiarity of the breast, and a hungry and irritable baby can calm down. The scenarios involving poor communication or infant distress may be endless and varied, but breastfeeding remains the same and provides parents a consistent way to communicate meaningfully and reassuringly with their young children.

EQUITABLE PARENTING

The ideal way to express parental love and concern is by breastfeeding babies on demand since frequent breastfeeding offers a great deal of human contact. As much as a baby receives oral nourishment from breastfeeding, a baby also learns at the breast that someone cares deeply about his well-being and his satisfaction. This person may be the breastfeeding mother, but she is representative of the family and the world at large. Only women can breastfeed, so the uniqueness of the womanly art of breastfeeding in child-rearing should be recognized widely.

In an effort to distribute infant care responsibilities more equitably, however, fathers are exhorted to feed young babies, even those who are breastfed exclusively. The feminist writer Peggy Orenstein offers this point of view in an interview conducted in *Parenting* magazine. Orenstein, who did not have children at the time of the interview, suggests the following in answer to the question of how mothers could get fathers more involved in infant care: "By letting dads spend time alone with their children from the beginning. If you're nursing, express milk, get out of the house, and leave your husband alone with the baby. When the baby cries while he's holding her, don't take her. Let him figure it out. Early on, it may feel good to be the only one who can calm the baby down, but if you start out this way, be prepared to still assume all the responsibility when the kid is 10 (Houppert 2000, 118)."

It may sound reasonable for Orenstein to suggest that a breastfeeding mother should take a break from baby care by pumping some milk and leaving her baby with the baby's father. This suggestion is both reckless and demeaning, however, when it is applied to a breastfeeding newborn or young baby. A breastfed baby, particularly during the early months of life, should be nursed at the breast. Only mothers can breastfeed, and instead of recognizing this unique role as an honorable responsibility, Orenstein views it as a burden.

Orenstein also imputes that a mother has to plan conscientiously for a father to take a much more active role early on in a baby's life, specifically by feeding the infant. She proposes interference with the breastfeeding dyad even though there are numerous ways in which a father can offer his assistance. For instance, a father can change a baby's diaper and clothes, cradle him, walk with him, talk to him, sit next to him, and simply be there for him. When the baby is six months old, a father can assist by preparing solid food and feeding the baby. Orenstein nevertheless suggests that unless fathers participate in infant feeding from early infancy, babies will forever remain bound only to their mothers. She even threatens, perhaps jokingly or not, that breastfeeding mothers will have to shoulder total responsibility for their children at the ripe age of ten years.

At best, Orenstein has a limited understanding of breastfeeding. First of all, a baby who nurses at the breast learns to relate not only to his breastfeeding mother but to his father, the rest of his family, and all other human beings. Second, at ten years of age children who have received the nurturing of breastfeeding are remarkably poised, cooperative, independent, and capable of thinking for themselves. Third, instead of permitting a father's role in a child's life to evolve naturally, Orenstein recommends an approach that would force a father to participate actively in early infant feeding and child care even though he is not equipped with the breasts that could so easily assuage an unhappy baby.

I offer criticism of Orenstein's advice specifically because her scenario includes a breastfed baby. Obviously, Orenstein appreciates the importance of breastfeeding, but it appears that she is unaware of the profound importance of breastfeeding as a holistic parenting activity. If her scenario had included a bottle-fed baby, it would be difficult to argue that there is a vast difference between a father feeding the baby versus a mother feeding the baby. In the case of infant formula-fed babies, fathers can surely participate more readily in early infant feeding. This cannot be said of breastfed babies, however, since there is no reason to subject a non-breastfeeding parent to the travails of consoling a baby who needs to breastfeed (although unforeseen circumstances may arise and lead to unexpected situations).

A good example of the type of anguish a father may experience when he is burdened with significant responsibility in infant care is presented by a psychiatrist in his parenting book. He was left alone with his six-month-old baby while his wife went out, and he describes the intense rage he felt at being unable to console his crying baby. Nothing he did comforted the baby, and his emotions far transcended exasperation: he was outraged and could barely control his anger. Years afterward the author is able to reflect upon this experience in order to make sense of his situation. He traces the anger back to his days as a pediatric intern when he had to inflict suffering upon crying young babies by performing medical procedures.

Understandably, such events occur as a matter of course in parenting. What is worrisome is that the guidance that is offered in parenting magazines, such as Orenstein's advice for fathers to participate actively and assertively in early child care, will actually increase the likelihood that more fathers will experience such exasperation and frustration with their infants. It is not at all clear to me that such suffering benefits either parent or infant.

As the movement to encourage fathers to participate more conscientiously in early infant care grows, true appreciation of the womanly art of breastfeeding may be further impeded. It does not help that pediatricians often undermine women's breastfeeding efforts in order to include fathers in early infant care. At well-baby check-ups, pediatricians may advise fathers to bottle-feed young infants, even those who are exclusively breastfed. Paternal participation in early infant care is both important and wonderful, but it should not interfere with breastfeeding.

At some point, it must be recognized that a mother's role is not the same as a father's role when it comes to dispensing care for young babies. A father's role may be supportive and helpful in infancy whereas the breastfeeding role of a mother is crucial. Both roles, however, are important in child-rearing. A father's role and a mother's role may be different, but they are mutually supportive and aimed toward the goal of best assuring the well-being of their baby.

SHARED INTIMACY

As a rule, a healthy breastfeeding relationship should not be interrupted so that a father may introduce a bottle of expressed breast milk or infant formula through a rubber nipple. Such interference may result in nipple confusion and the devaluation of a woman's unique role in her baby's life. Instead of viewing breastfeeding as a mere source of breast milk, it should be considered as an activity that encompasses the well-being of the entire young human being whose life begins as a baby.

Breastfeeding benefits all young children, including those who have congenital disorders. For instance, Arlene Jacobs recounts the brief life of her young baby who was born with Severe Combined Immune Deficiency, a rare condition that left her baby unable to develop immunity to infection. He remained healthy during the first four and a half months of life when he was exclusively breastfed. After he was exposed to eating solid food, he developed hives that cleared once he returned to exclusive breastfeeding.

At six months of age, however, her baby began experiencing repeated infections. A bone marrow transplant was performed when he was nine months old, and he died of complications from the transplant at eighteen months of age. Jacobs (1997, 34) summarizes the impact breastfeeding had upon her son's short life: "My breastmilk kept him healthy for the first six months of his life. My breastmilk kept him alive for 18 months." The power of breastfeeding to improve the quality of life for all babies should not be taken lightly.

A breastfed baby receives ideal nourishment, special protection against germs, growth factors that stimulate healthy development, warmth, touch, love, and his mother's presence. From the newborn period onward, a baby can be nourished at the breast with optimal nutrition and protective substances that can shield the baby from infection and illness. As the baby receives the warm nourishment of customized breast milk, he can also touch and feel the warmth of his mother's living skin. After his little body is sated with breast milk, he can rest; most babies, in fact, are content and relaxed enough to fall asleep at the breast.

Dissenters who opine that the act of bottle-feeding is the same as breastfeeding generally ignore the fact that the physical intimacy of breastfeeding cannot easily be replicated with bottle-feeding. Although it is possible for a mother to bare her breast and abdomen so that a bottle-fed baby can explore his mother's skin and receive some tactile stimulation, few mothers would even think of doing this. Additionally, Ashley Montagu (1986, 83) notes that since babies suckle at both breasts, nurslings receive stimulation to both sides of their faces and bodies as they breastfeed.

In contrast, bottle-fed babies are usually cradled in the same position at every feeding. A right-handed parent, for instance, will probably feel more comfortable cradling the baby in her left arm while holding the bottle in her right hand. Moreover, many parents enjoy seeing their babies feed themselves, so it is not uncommon for young babies to hold their own bottles or lie down with bottles propped up and held to their mouths. Regardless of how lovingly parents offer their babies bottles of infant formula, the act of bottle-feeding cannot provide the intimacy that nursing at the breast provides.

Although the vast majority of bottle-feeding parents attend with care to the details of properly preparing, storing, and warming infant formula for their babies, there may be unusual cases in which parents can demonstrate willful negligence and perhaps cruelty. My sister, for example, knew a couple in New York who insisted on feeding their young infant daughter cold infant formula straight from the refrigerator in the middle of the winter. The bottle-fed baby had no choice but to drink what was offered. My sister tried to convince the baby's father that the infant formula should be warmed, but he merely laughed at her suggestion.

ON DEMAND BREASTFEEDING

When parents breastfeed on demand, they do not have to think about their baby's needs in ways that bottle-feeding parents do. For example, nursing at the breast would not expose a baby to drinking cold milk. Breast milk is composed of fluid, substances, and cells that are produced by a living mother's body. The secretion of breast milk at body temperature ensures the breastfed baby the delivery of a dynamic fluid that contains bioactive components.

Since breast milk will generally be available once the milk has come in and the breastfeeding relationship has been established, one rarely needs to worry about running out of milk. Economists have remarked that breastfeeding offers a model example of the theory of supply and demand: demand drives the supply such that increased suckling at the breast will increase production of the milk supply. Moreover, breast milk is always prepared freshly without preservatives or additives, so it provides truly unprocessed and unadulterated nourishment.

Once the art of breastfeeding is learned, many women learn how simple childrearing can be. For far too long, however, women have been misinformed that breastfeeding is optional and only for babies under the age of six months. Even though the American Academy of Pediatrics (AAP) now advocates a minimum of one year of breastfeeding, some pediatricians still do not comprehend why a baby should be breastfed for more than six months.

As most breastfeeding parents already know, pediatricians possess their own opinions about breastfeeding. For example, a respected and popular Los Angeles pediatrician told my friend that her six-month-old son did not need to breastfeed. He told her confidentially, "After six months, breastfeeding's just for the mother." In New York, my sister had a similar experience with her baby's pediatrician. At her baby's well-child check-ups, the pediatrician expressed surprise every time my sister reported that she was breastfeeding her infant son, even when he was only a few months old. Pediatricians often bias their advice according to whether or not they understand or appreciate the benefits of breastfeeding.

Fortunately, a small but growing number of pediatricians have become more vocal in their advocacy of breastfeeding. Knowledgeable pediatricians are speaking out so that correct information about breastfeeding can be given to parents. In the twenty-first century, it is a novel idea that pediatricians should dispense accurate and positive information about breastfeeding to the parents of their young patients.

Breastfeeding is an intimate and interactive activity that draws a mother closely to her child. From the newborn period onward, the young nursling needs to breastfeed as often as every one to three hours around the clock since human milk is easily digestible. The quick digestion of human milk is ideal from every medical perspective because it suits perfectly the immature digestive tract of the newborn and young baby. Also, frequent nursing provides the baby with a constant supply of fresh nutrients and factors for healthy growth and development.

Women may be concerned that they will not produce enough breast milk, but frequent nursing should generate milk plentifully. In cultures such as the !Kung San, mothers are with their babies almost constantly because breastfeeding is valued so highly. Hence, these mothers encourage their babies to breastfeed often and on demand.

In Western culture, where breastfeeding is not popular, babies are often kept at arm's length, and most mothers do not encourage their babies to breastfeed often. It is important, however, to permit a baby to breastfeed throughout the day and night as needed. Although breastfeeding mothers may fear frequent nursing during the night, most will adapt to nighttime nursing without too much difficulty.

NIGHTTIME NURSING

The majority of young babies do not sleep through the night, but parents will invariably hear stories about babies who began sleeping through the night immediately. It is natural for parents to dread interrupted nighttime sleep and hope that their baby will sleep through the night. After all, it is exhausting to merely contemplate the idea of getting up several times a night to nurse or offer a bottle to a baby. Consequently, parents may look for easy solutions when it comes to dealing with the nighttime feeding patterns of their young babies.

Most parenting books advise parents to approach nighttime feedings in a business-like manner so that babies do not enjoy nighttime feedings. Parents are discouraged from talking to their babies, rocking their babies, and interacting too lovingly with their babies. This type of parental detachment is supposed to encourage babies to go right back to the business of sleeping so that parents can also return to sleep quickly.

It is reasonable to sympathize with sleep deprived parents, but there is something amiss with advice that urges inconsistency on the part of parents' behavior toward their young babies. It is unreasonable for a parent to be loving and responsive during the daytime and then distant and nearly unresponsive late at night. Granted, parents have no need to be unnaturally cheerful and enthusiastic in the middle of the night to greet a hungry infant. There is nothing at all wrong nevertheless with offering a crying and hungry baby some soft caresses of love and a few words of affection. Parents should be able to provide a nurturing response to their babies' needs regardless of the time.

Breastfeeding satisfies a baby's hunger, and it also encourages both mother and baby to slumber off to sleep peacefully. The latter effect is accomplished via the influence of endorphins, which are neurotransmitters that are known to suppress pain and induce pleasure (Odent 1994). Breastfeeding stimulates the production and release of endorphins into both the mother's bloodstream and breast milk. Irrespective of the time of day, breastfeeding is a physiologically complex activity that helps to ensure the well-being of the nursing dyad.

In the early weeks of a baby's life, a mother may even appreciate the opportunity to see her baby in the middle of the night regardless of the time. She might feel energetic because she is in love with her baby, or she might simply want to reassure herself that her baby is fine. When a mother follows her intuition and listens to her young baby, she will fear neither her baby's needs nor her own need to respond to her baby.

In reality, a mother has a biological need to respond to her baby's various needs by breastfeeding, even in the middle of the night. As mentioned earlier, breastfeeding benefits both infant and mother. There is no reason to distinguish the needs of a baby from the needs of his mother as if they are mutually exclusive. Although it may be true that a mother will sleep through the night if she is given the opportunity, her body still needs to recover from pregnancy and childbirth. As much as a baby may need to breastfeed, a mother also needs to breastfeed since it may take weeks or even months for her uterus to return to its normal size.

Regardless of the health benefits breastfeeding provides, some parents may use infant formula since formula-fed babies tend to sleep for longer stretches of time than do breastfed babies. In truth, if adults ingested a large amount of barely digestible food like infant formula, they would probably be sleepy as well. Parents should, however, consider whether or not the possible gain of a few hours' sleep by using infant formula is worth the risk of perhaps disrupting a lifetime's worth of long-term health benefits gained by breastfeeding.

Instead of viewing breastfeeding as an unnecessary and inconvenient activity, it should be appreciated for the highly complex process it is. Breastfeeding works best when a mother is available to offer breast milk as frequently as possible. In order to produce an abundant supply of breast milk, the breasts need to be suckled frequently and consistently around the clock. Once they are adequately stimulated, breasts will produce milk on demand. Additionally, when mothers empty their full breasts, their chances of experiencing engorgement and its complications will decrease.

CO-SLEEPING

By sleeping together in the same bed, or co-sleeping, a baby is kept close to her mother at nighttime. Co-sleeping facilitates breastfeeding since a mother does not need to get out of bed in order to heat up infant formula while her baby cries with hunger and discomfort. The breast, if offered, will be able to nourish and comfort a baby all through the night while causing minimal inconvenience for either mother or father.

The American Academy of Pediatrics (2005) offers the following guidance to parents and physicians: "Mother and infant should sleep in proximity to each other to facilitate breastfeeding." This is a bold statement because many parents and physicians are either unfamiliar with the idea of babies sleeping near their parents or they are opposed to the practice.

Although there have been a small number of unusual cases in which parents accidentally smothered their infants by co-sleeping, the choice to co-sleep involves common sense. Parents who take rigorous and sound measures to ensure the safety of their sleeping infants will be able to reap the benefits of co-sleeping. This means, naturally, that parents will not indulge in the use of alcohol or illicit drugs, or in any way endanger the infants who sleep in their beds.

There are some parents and physicians, however, who fear that parents will either err or cause intentional mischief. Such fears engender a blanket condemnation of co-sleeping, which is terribly unfortunate. The vast majority of healthy and sensible parents use common sense, and they care deeply about the well-being of their young infants. Those parents who think they may possibly harm their babies should not attempt to co-sleep. Co-sleeping, however, has been a worldwide practice among human beings throughout history. Parents who wish to co-sleep with their infants should feel confident that scrupulous attention to their young infants' well-being and safety in their beds will yield greater nighttime comfort and ease of mind for the entire family.

FORCED DETACHMENT

Some parents, however, are unwilling or possibly afraid to accommodate the needs of their young infants whether it is daytime or nighttime. The prevailing parenting culture tends to promote detachment, separation, avoidance, and distance instead of intimacy, physical closeness, and availability. In this type of parenting atmosphere, it is no wonder that parents choose consciously, however unwillingly sometimes, to ignore their babies' needs. Hence, many parents are willing to let their babies cry for prolonged periods of time, especially at nighttime. Although it is difficult for parents to endure their babies' crying, the majority will keep the doors closed and let their babies cry alone and unattended.

Breastfeeding on demand, on the other hand, obliterates the need for babies to cry themselves to sleep alone. Breastfeeding easily comforts and satisfies hungry babies; it provides parents a tool to interact effectively with their needy babies. Regrettably, many parents misunderstand breastfeeding and mistrust their own intuition. This is the case since parents are routinely advised that they will spoil their babies if they respond too efficiently or too lovingly to their babies' needs.

Sadly, a most prevalent view of a young baby's needs is that the experience of frustration will strengthen her character and teach her that life is not always gratifying. It is peculiar that such a view of a baby's ability to learn could be promulgated in light of how parents often disregard a young baby's mental and emotional growth and development. In fact, millions of parents actually trust that any care is satisfactory for their babies as long as it is safe, clean, and somewhat educational. This means, obviously, that parents do not think much real development is occurring in the minds and hearts of their little babies. The same parents, however, expect their babies to somehow learn that their needs should not and will not always be satisfied. Ultimately, there is an inherent contradiction in the way many parents understand their babies' capacity to learn.

Parents may think that they are teaching their babies some form of discipline by delaying satisfaction of their babies' need for nourishment, comfort, touch, or love. Early infancy, however, is not at all the time for parents to demand disciplined behavior since babies cannot control their biological needs. If parents choose to persist in teaching lessons to their babies early in life, the result will more likely be that young infants will learn to experience frustration repeatedly. Eventually, these babies might learn a great deal about disappointment and distress while they learn little about the meaning of cooperation and satisfaction.

There is something terribly wrong when parents are advised to deny babies the fundamental right to be cared for with love and responsiveness. The advice parents should be receiving is that they should attach themselves to their babies and nurture the ability to comfort their babies as no one else can. If babies wake up often through the night, then parents can try to help the babies they have brought into this world. Whether it is daytime or nighttime, a breastfeeding mother can provide for her baby uniquely maternal and consistently loving, caring, affectionate, and powerfully nourishing human interaction.

LOVE AND COOPERATION AT THE BREAST

Young children learn the significance of love and cooperation from the repeated experience of receiving satisfaction of their basic needs. As discussed earlier, there is nothing abstract about a baby's need to be nourished; to love and be loved; and to be cared for, held, and carried. These needs are real, and their satisfaction through breastfeeding constitutes the essence of healthy human development.

Breastfeeding satisfies most young children's needs because it offers affection, concern, discipline, dedication, and consistency. These are the same human attributes that exemplify and promote both love and cooperation. When young children receive the myriad benefits of breastfeeding, the task of parenting is what it should be: it is a natural and effective form of communication between parents and their children.

As mentioned earlier, breastfeeding can offer young children succor even when mothers may not necessarily be in loving moods. Also, since moods are transient, a mother may experience a positive transformation of her mood while she breastfeeds. Over the course of six years, I breastfed two children and experienced the wonders of meaningful human interaction. Breastfeeding humanized me and taught me a great deal about the significance of love, cooperation, consideration, warmth, and touch. Similarly, breastfeeding instilled in the lives of my children a profound understanding of and appreciation for love and cooperation.

One cannot expect children to learn how to love and be loved if they are not given the opportunity to learn from a consistently available and loving caregiver. It is difficult for babies and children to develop humane social values if they cannot repeatedly interact with and observe the example of caring, loving, and available parents. From this perspective, a mother's love and breastfeeding will most likely serve as the most secure foundation for a young child's healthy existence.

MATERNAL AVAILABILITY

It is important and possible for women to care for young children during the formative years. Women can surely return to work outside the home when their children no longer need constant maternal care. Women today live longer, and the average woman can expect to live well into her seventies. During such a long lifetime, there will be numerous opportunities for women to demonstrate their intelligence, beauty, uniqueness, talents, and strengths.

Grandma Moses can serve as a good role model for women who think that success and fame in life can only be secured while they are young or relatively young. Grandma Moses' art was displayed at the San Diego Museum of Art in 2001, and the museum offered the following biographical information: Grandma Moses began painting at the age of 75, gained renown for her naïve art, lived until the age of 101 years, painted nearly 1,600 paintings, and achieved long-lasting fame. Grandma Moses' prolific career demonstrates how much women can achieve in life beyond the childbearing years and through old age. In other words, there is little need for women to become supermoms.

Indeed, it might be better for the general public to marvel at a few women celebrities and other ambitious women as they become supermoms. Celebrities can become pregnant, bear babies, remain fit, earn large sums of money, grace magazine covers, and enjoy stardom. Similarly, business executives and professionals can work long hours, have children, exercise regularly, socialize, and earn suitable amounts of money. It is evident that there will always be some women who can do many things well simultaneously. At the same time, there are different ways to live, and not all women or men wish or need to strive to succeed at the level that the media and contemporary culture hype as being admirable.

In the modern era, one of the biggest challenges that must be confronted is the failure to recognize the importance of both parental love and hands-on maternal care to the well-being of young children. The psychologist Isabelle Fox writes in *Being There: The Benefits of a Stay-at-Home Parent* that the frequent absence of parental care in her patients' histories often impairs her ability to help children in her clinical practice. Many of Fox's patients are troubled children and adolescents who do not have recollections of early childhood experiences that might have contributed to the subsequent development of mental or emotional problems. Unfortunately, many of these patients' parents are similarly clueless since they relegated their children's care to nannies or day care settings.

Fox advises parents to be more available and try to stay home with their children during the formative years. Fox happens to treat young patients who live in the wealthier enclaves of Los Angeles, but psychiatric problems arise irrespective of wealth or social status. Regardless of the intelligence or success of her patients' parents, there are no guarantees that any child can be assured of sound mental health. If parents wish to understand why their children grow and develop as they do, then parents need to be more available during their children's formative years since it takes time and effort to nurture children's sound mental health.

THE TABOO OF BREASTFEEDING

It may sometimes be difficult for a woman to even mention that she is breastfeeding because many people misunderstand this art and practice. I have a friend who was sporadically breastfeeding her three-year-old daughter when she moved into a typical middle-class suburban community. After a few months of befriending her neighbors, my friend revealed unintentionally to her next-door neighbor that she was still occasionally breastfeeding her daughter. The neighbor, the mother of two non-breastfed toddlers, withdrew her friendship; within three months the neighbor had sold her house and moved into another house in the same community. My friend's experience is not atypical. Breastfeeding is so misunderstood that women are rarely seen breastfeeding in public.

In recent years some nursing mothers have been trying actively to make it easier for women to breastfeed in public. Amy Harmon reports in the June 7, 2005, issue of the *New York Times* that Barbara Walters, the television host and celebrity, mentioned on her show *The View* that she felt uncomfortable sitting next to a breastfeeding woman. In response to her nationally broadcast comment, approximately 200 breastfeeding mothers gathered outside Walters' office in Manhattan the next morning and held their babies and signs in support of breastfeeding. These women, also known as "lactivists," are trying to encourage women to breastfeed in public.

When breastfeeding mothers are among like-minded individuals who also appreciate the importance of breastfeeding, it becomes that much easier to breastfeed without inhibition. About nine years ago, when I was home schooling my son I joined a small home schooling group in my area. We visited together at local parks, and I met women who were breastfeeding toddlers and pre-schoolers. We breastfed our children at the park, and we talked openly and comfortably about child-rearing, breastfeeding, and education.

Whereas a supportive environment encourages breastfeeding, an unsupportive environment achieves the opposite and dissuades many women from breastfeeding. I once met a woman whose family had gone on a cruise when her baby was ten months old. The woman's elder sister, a childless physician in her late twenties, was averse to breastfeeding and expressed contempt whenever the baby nursed. The sister created such a hostile environment that the woman weaned her baby off the breast.

Undoubtedly, the woman had been intimidated by her ignorant but accomplished and highly educated sister. When the woman learned that my eighteen-month-old daughter was breastfeeding, she tried valiantly to nurse her son since he had been weaned off the breast only a month earlier. He seemed confused, so she did not pursue breastfeeding any further.

One must have fortitude and conviction to withstand the criticism that will come from those who are unaware of what breastfeeding offers. Even though this mother knew how much breastfeeding meant to her baby since he was thriving, she did not have the confidence to dismiss her sister's uninformed bias against breastfeeding. When others fail to comprehend the benefits of breastfeeding, the best one can do is to show the actual proof of one's parenting philosophy in one's own life.

REJECTION OF THE BREAST

There may come a time when a breastfeeding baby suddenly rejects the breast. An exclusively breastfed baby under the age of six months should not refuse the breast if the breast is her only source of nourishment. Parents should consider seeking medical advice if the baby rejects the breast repeatedly, and she is behaving differently. For the majority of breastfed babies who are ingesting other food or liquid, however, it is possible that a baby may reject the breast on a temporary basis.

Although many parents perceive a baby's rejection of the breast to be a definitive sign that she has had her fill of breastfeeding, a baby may have numerous reasons for rejecting the breast temporarily. She may not feel well, her appetite may be diminished, she may have lost a little interest in nursing, the breast milk may taste different (particularly when nursing mothers become pregnant), or she may simply not wish to breastfeed. Regardless of the causes behind the rejection of the breast, a baby should not be weaned off the breast when her interest in breastfeeding decreases.

The reality is that a baby may lose her appetite for breastfeeding just as an older child may lose her appetite for food. No one, however, would suggest denying an older child food in the future; if anything, the child would be encouraged to consume more food. In contrast, the baby who rejects the breast is treated differently. It is assumed automatically that breastfeeding should cease, and that the baby will easily survive without breastfeeding. Thus, a baby who rejects the breast even on a temporary basis is immediately perceived to have outgrown breastfeeding.

When my daughter was ten months old, we experienced one day when she did not wish to breastfeed. Since my son had breastfed non-stop for nearly three years, I could not understand why my daughter would wish to stop at ten months. It did not make sense to me, and I knew how important breastfeeding was in our lives. Therefore, I persisted in offering my daughter the breast throughout that day, and she continued to reject it. By the next day, she resumed nursing as if she had never stopped, and she continued until she was nearly three years old.

Instead of supposing that a baby has lost complete interest in breastfeeding, a mother should keep encouraging her baby to nurse. By continuing to offer the breast, a mother extols the value of breastfeeding, and the baby will learn that breastfeeding is important enough to be resumed. Most babies who are breastfed on demand without artificial milk substitutes will recommence breastfeeding if they are encouraged to do so. In such cases, a mother's availability is crucial to resuming breastfeeding.

ACCESSIBLE NURTURING

When my son was six years old, his closest friend's mother was often preoccupied with her house renovation, volunteering at her son's school, and her social life. All my son's friend knew about domestic life was that his mother was busy shopping and decorating their home while the housekeeper took care of him and his younger brother. In the meantime, this little boy always saw me with my children, and he did not see a housekeeper when he visited our apartment.

The little boy was flabbergasted since I did the cleaning and cooking, and my husband and I did not use babysitters. He was unaccustomed to the concept of hands-on maternal care. We eventually lost touch with this boy and his family, but I learned later that this boy is troubled and has experienced terrible problems in school. Although his family maintains a wealthy lifestyle, it seems to lack substance and humanity.

By making myself available to my children, particularly by breastfeeding on demand, our children received a most profound and meaningful foundation in life that is based upon satisfaction, love, comfort, warmth, intimacy, open communication, cooperation, and sharing. Both children are deeply connected not only to my thoughts, my sense of humor (or lack thereof), my emotions, and my life but most certainly to their father as well. They adore their father, and they appreciate him greatly.

Several years ago, I pursued a less than enlightened train of thought when I became bewildered by the marvelous rapport our children had with my husband. I wondered if my children would have been close to us even if I had not stayed home all these years. I realized, after overcoming my bout of jealousy, how utterly wrong it was to begrudge our children's attachment to their father. The children's intimate connection to their father was, after all, the greatest evidence that breastfeeding enhances a child's relationship not only to the nursing mother but most certainly to the father as well.

When a baby is breastfed on demand, she learns that someone loves her, cares for her, responds to her, and cooperates with her. The lessons learned at the breast form a sound foundation upon which a baby can then establish healthy relationships with other human beings later in life. A baby's ability to learn the rudiments of meaningful and loving social behavior should not be underestimated. In fact, the lessons are learned so well that young children can become the greatest teachers.

My daughter, for instance, has always been my son's greatest defender. Even as a baby, she would cry in sympathy if I scolded my son. As a little toddler, she would walk up to her brother if he was crying, and she would dry his tears. After she started speaking, she would come over to tell me that it was not nice of me to yell at her brother. My daughter's ability to communicate her sympathy toward her brother helped me to reflect upon my behavior. There were times when I had no idea how overwrought I had become over some minor incident, but a little touch from my daughter's small hand would help to bring me back in touch with my humanity.

When young children experience healthy satisfaction of basic physical and emotional needs early in life, they can do more than survive and adapt to varying environmental circumstances. Young children can even improve the state of humanity and offer the goodness of their loving hearts to the adults labeled by Ashley Montagu to be "adulterated children."

To this day, my children teach me how to be happy, and I can hardly offer them enough gratitude for giving me the opportunity to reflect upon my own actions. I can bestow kisses and hugs nearly constantly, and it is amazing to think that these two children were nurtured by a fairly cold fish like me. The healthy nurturing of our humanity, particularly mine, was bolstered greatly by breastfeeding.

7

THE CULTURE OF BREASTFEEDING

COMFORT AND PROTECTION

I am thankful that my children breastfed for nearly three years each. When my son was almost three years old, my obstetrician recommended that I stop nursing my son. He feared that nipple stimulation would precipitate the onset of preterm labor during my second pregnancy. It turned out that I had preterm labor even though I stopped nursing my son.

Before my daughter's third birthday, I learned to my embarrassment and dismay that she had two cavities. I was guilt-ridden since I had not been cleaning her teeth diligently enough; I acceded readily to the dentist's assessment that my daughter no longer needed to nurse. With my approval, the dentist gently lectured my daughter to stop nursing, and she stopped breastfeeding that day.

Unfortunately, in the absence of breastfeeding, my daughter suffered with frequent respiratory infections and repeated ear infections. Whenever she caught a cold, she became pale, and she was visibly weakened by her infection. Whereas she had never exhibited such signs while she was breastfed, it was clear that her immunity had become compromised once she stopped breastfeeding.

Even though my daughter had experienced her share of upper respiratory infections as an infant and toddler, she never had an ear infection. While she was breastfed on demand for the first three years of her life, she suffered minimally from her colds. If she became sick, she lost little sleep at night, experienced crankiness rarely, and continued to breastfeed as usual.

My daughter benefited immensely from breastfeeding: not only was she protected from acquiring serious infectious illnesses but she was easily comforted by breastfeeding. Undoubtedly, this was the case since breast milk contains endorphins, which are natural hormones that suppress pain. Breastfeeding provides a nursing child both hormone-mediated comfort and the presence of an available and loving caregiver.

Our lives were simplified dramatically throughout the years my children were breastfed. In 1995, for instance, we took a cross-country airplane flight even though I was not well. On the morning of our departure, I had a mild sore throat, and our two-year-old daughter had a fever. I asked her repeatedly if she wanted to go to New York, and she responded negatively each time. Since we had non-refundable airplane tickets I did not wish to waste, I wound up convincing myself and my two-year-old that we should go on the trip.

As the morning progressed, I felt increasingly worse while my daughter felt better. I was ill by the time we boarded the airplane: my ears were plugged, I had difficulty hearing, and my sore throat had become painful. During the airplane ride, I tried to sleep off the discomfort while my husband took care of our children. Our daughter was comfortable in her father's arms, and my husband simply handed her over to me whenever she needed to nurse. Despite the rapid deterioration of my own health, breastfeeding provided me with a resource to comfort my nursing toddler.

Most non-breastfeeding parents rarely have a comparably effective tool with which to comfort their young babies and children. For instance, I once examined a little two-year-old patient at the office for his regular check-up. Toward the end of the visit, his mother gave me a pleading look and asked if there was anything I could prescribe in order to get her son to sleep on the airplane.

This was a wonderful and loving mother who dreaded the cross-country trip from Los Angeles to New York with her toddler. Frankly, she wanted me to prescribe a sedative. I was thoroughly surprised by her request and unprepared to respond, so I consulted with my colleague. Parents had been asking him the same question over the many years of his medical practice, and he simply recommended an over-the-counter anti-histamine that offers the side effect of drowsiness.

Few parents are aware of the enormous secondary benefits of breastfeeding, particularly its ability to soothe and comfort young children. Throughout early childhood, there are numerous situations in which young babies and children need comfort and reassurance. Breastfeeding provides consistency in a young child's life when so much else can be new and strange. Clearly, breastfeeding is not simply oral nutrition for young babies.

The American Academy of Pediatrics (AAP) now recommends that babies be breastfed for at least one year, and the World Health Organization (WHO) advises a minimum of two years (WHO 2004). Even so, over one-third of American newborns are not breastfed at all, and only 12 percent are breastfed for one year. The prevalent understanding of breastfeeding is that any amount of breastfeeding, even if it occurs only during the immediate newborn period, is sufficient.

PROLONGED BREASTFEEDING

Anthropologist Katherine Dettwyler (1995, 39) used nonhuman primate breastfeeding patterns to predict that the age of weaning for children should be between 2.5 and 7 years. By examining the weaning ages of primate species like the chimpanzees and the gorillas, she determined several factors that influence natural weaning. Although some pediatricians suggest that human infants should nurse as long as the human gestation, which is approximately nine months, Dettwyler's research showed that chimpanzees and gorillas nurse their babies for six times the length of gestation. Accordingly, human beings should breastfeed for about 4.5 years.

Other pediatricians use the guideline of tripling a baby's birth weight to determine the length of breastfeeding, which often results in the discontinuation of breastfeeding at about one year of age. In contrast, Dettwyler (1995, 46) notes that larger mammals nurse their babies until they have quadrupled their birth weight. Quadrupling of birth weight in human beings occurs at about 2.5 to 3.5 years of age. Citing other studies of natural weaning ages for primates, Dettwyler advocates a minimum of 2.5 years of breastfeeding for children.

Such a view of breastfeeding and weaning will surprise the majority of parents and health practitioners. Since the culture of bottle-feeding has become so pervasive, the subject of weaning from the breast is rarely broached. After all, how many women breastfeed their babies beyond a few weeks or several months?

When my children agreed to stop breastfeeding, I was initially relieved because I thought nearly three years each was sufficient. In both cases, I was influenced by the advice of other health practitioners. I was an educated pediatrician who appreciated breastfeeding's benefits, but I acquiesced when my obstetrician and the children's dentist questioned my children's need to breastfeed.

I mentioned earlier my daughter's repeated bouts with infection, but equally terrible was the emotional trauma my son experienced when I stopped breastfeeding him. Around the time that my son stopped breastfeeding at the age of three years, I began to push him toward greater independence. Part of this mind-set was due to the ill health and discomfort that accompanied my second pregnancy. After my daughter's birth, I was convinced that I could not handle sleeping with two children. Therefore, I asked my son to sleep with his father in a separate bed while I nursed his sister and slept with her. I effectively rejected my son without understanding how emotionally bereft he felt.

My mother was visiting at the time of my daughter's birth, and she warned me that my son needed more attention. She advised that the least I should do was to continue to let him sleep with me. Instead, I complained that I had already given him so much of my attention, that he was getting bigger, and that he could handle the change. He was, after all, a whopping three years old. I write this facetiously because when I look at photographs of my three-year-old, all I see is a small, young child who deserved more attention than I gave him. In other words, I expected too much of my son once he turned three years old.

The glaring mistake I made was to presume that my three-year-old was ready to become independent of me. In many ways, the end of breastfeeding signaled a period of transition for me and my son, but it was not necessarily fulfilling for either of us. I assumed wrongly that three years of breastfeeding would be the greatest foundation for his security and well-being. In truth, I could have offered him much more.

If I had perhaps not convinced myself that he had slept long enough with me at nighttime, then I might have diminished his misery. Instead, he shouldered a succession of burdens that I imposed upon him: he needed to cease breastfeeding, welcome the birth of a baby sister, and tolerate my abrupt one-sided decision for him to sleep with his father after having always slept with both of us. All of this caused my young son confusion.

One cannot suppose unequivocally that a three-year-old child is ready to wean from the breast and declare his independence from his mother. Although the vast majority of babies are not breastfed today, this does not mean that even three years of breastfeeding is sufficient or too much. A child should be given the opportunity to breastfeed for as long as he needs. After all, one cannot presume to know a child's needs if one fails to look at the child's needs in the first place.

The fact is that young children are needy and helpless, and there is no magic age at which those needs suddenly disappear. My error was to take for granted my three-year-old son's ability to continue exhibiting kindness, love, cooperation, and patience when I did not display similar behavior. Before his sister's birth he did little wrong because I had patience and the ability to communicate. After her birth, however, I started to become impatient with my toddler because I changed my expectations of him. Whereas he ordinarily felt free to be himself, I suddenly began to expect a great deal from him. It was as if I believed that three years of breastfeeding was all I had to do for him, and he would be nearly perfect.

Admittedly, I had become a bit fixated with the idea of three years of breastfeeding, and I seemed to have forgotten about the meaning of unconditional love and gentle patience. When I stopped breastfeeding my three-year-old son, I was convinced that I had given him enough of my time, my love, and my dedication. Like many parents who complain bitterly that they give so much to their children and receive so little in return, I began to misconstrue my young son's immaturity. As a toddler he was no longer totally helpless, but he was still in need of assistance on occasion. Instead of offering consistent kindness, consideration, and sympathy, I sometimes became cold, demanding, and insensitive.

For instance, many years ago I raced through a mall as I pushed my daughter in her stroller and expected my small four-year-old son to run behind me. I was distraught and nervous because we were late meeting my husband for lunch. We had three more blocks to walk, and I was walking much too quickly. Suddenly, my son fell, and he landed on his hands and knees. I looked at him, and all I thought was that he was delaying me. Instead of making sure he was all right and offering a kind word, I ordered him to get up and keep moving. Nearby, a young woman looked at me and muttered aloud, "What a bitch!" She was right.

The reality was that I could have easily done several things to alter the hectic nature of my situation. Instead, I put my son in a vulnerable position and, naturally, he fell. When I scolded my son for delaying us, he could only respond in disbelief as he observed my nervous and flustered behavior. He had rarely experienced such an onslaught of negativity from me while he was breastfed.

Breastfeeding had offered my son a consistent source of affection, love, security, and assurance. As long as I was breastfeeding him, I remained closely connected to him and intimately aware of his needs. Once he stopped breastfeeding, however, I became less attuned to his needs. Whereas I rarely had to think consciously about how to nurture my son while I was breastfeeding him, I now had to face the challenge of communicating with him without the touch of breastfeeding.

In other words, I was able to easily communicate my unconditional love to my son while I was breastfeeding him. He knew that I was there for him, loved him, was interested in his well-being, and was concerned about him. All this and more I could transmit easily through breastfeeding. In fact, I rarely had to put complete conscious effort into nursing either of my children.

Much like the phenomenon of pregnancy, wherein a life develops within one's womb without much conscious input, breastfeeding also enables a life to develop at one's breast in a similar way. This is not to say that breastfeeding is a mindless activity. Rather, it seems to be a truism that life is often simpler when one puts less conscious thought into what one does. This is certainly the case with breastfeeding since more mothers would probably enjoy it if they thought less about it.

BREASTFEEDING AT LARGE

In recent years more American women from all walks of life have begun to breastfeed their babies. This trend is worthy of the highest praise since breastfeeding benefits mothers, their babies, families, and society at large. It is discouraging to note, however, that women sometimes breastfeed without receiving sufficient knowledgeable support from their spouses, family members, medical practitioners, or friends. As a rule, women can breastfeed successfully if they are well-informed and determined to breastfeed. There are exceptions, sadly, when a lack of education, opportunity, or wisdom undermines a woman's sincerest efforts to succeed with breastfeeding.

Several years ago there was a widely publicized case in which a young mother in New York was tried for manslaughter and convicted of criminally negligent homicide in the death of her breastfed infant son. Tabitha Walrond was an unmarried nineteen-year-old black welfare recipient whose seven-week-old breastfed son died of dehydration and starvation: the baby weighed nearly three pounds less than he did at birth.

Tabitha Walrond was unlucky throughout her pregnancy and as a new mother. She was unable to schedule her newborn's check-up with a health practitioner because of poverty and repeated bureaucratic complications with paperwork for her baby's medical visits. At Walrond's post-partum check-up, according to an October 1, 1997, article by Rachel L. Swarns in the *New York Times*, a doctor noticed that the baby was thin, and he weighed the baby. The baby was noted to have gained two ounces, but he was not examined by a health practitioner.

Further complicating the situation was the estrangement of the baby's father from Walrond and the fact that he had originally wanted her to get an abortion. He did not see the baby until eight days before the baby's death. The baby's father worked later with the prosecutor to try to convict Walrond of manslaughter.

Nina Bernstein reports in the April 28, 1999, issue of the *New York Times* that Walrond underwent surgical breast reduction at the age of fifteen. She also gave birth via cesarean section and had complications with the surgery that required her to stop breastfeeding for several days. These various factors contributed significantly to Walrond's inability to nourish her son adequately at the breast.

Despite Walrond's significant medical and surgical history, however, hospital records show that she was discharged without receiving either advice for the potential problems she might encounter with breastfeeding or an appointment for her newborn's check-up at two weeks of age. In all probability, Walrond thought she would produce more than enough breast milk since she was originally endowed with an abundance of breast tissue. Instead, her endeavors to breastfeed turned out disastrously. A sincere but uneducated and poor young woman like Walrond, who thought she was doing her best for her baby, should not have been so isolated from the culture of breastfeeding.

RECENT ADVOCACY OF BREASTFEEDING

The American Academy of Pediatrics (AAP) has always supported breastfeeding, but for decades it advocated breastfeeding for only six months. It was not until December 1997 that the AAP issued a revised and comprehensive pro-breastfeeding policy statement. The AAP now recommends that babies be breastfed for at least one year with exclusive breastfeeding for the first six months of life.

Tabitha Walrond, an unemployed welfare recipient, was breastfeeding her son in the summer of 1997, at a time when many pediatricians were not necessarily supportive of women's efforts to breastfeed their babies. Also, as an indigent woman, Walrond challenged a reflexive infant feeding behavior among the poor by choosing to breastfeed and not to bottle-feed. Her unfortunate history and circumstances, sadly, led to a disastrous outcome.

Until recently, it was unusual for a woman on welfare assistance to breastfeed since the government-sponsored food program for indigent women and children, Supplemental Nutrition Program for Women, Infants and Children (WIC), has been promoting the free distribution of government-purchased infant formula for the past three decades. WIC was established originally to help poor women and their young children improve their nutritional and health status. One of the program's major outcomes, however, was the widespread use of infant formula among the poor.

WIC endorsed the use of infant formula for so long that it currently faces a significant challenge in trying to convince indigent women that they should be breastfeeding their newborns and infants. In contrast to the past practice of promoting infant formula use, WIC in various parts of the country is currently promoting breastfeeding actively. For instance, the California WIC upholds a breastfeeding mission statement that encourages women to breastfeed exclusively for the first six months and through the first year of infancy (California Dept. of Health Services 2005).

Nevertheless, despite an ongoing educational campaign by WIC to encourage and support breastfeeding, breastfeeding rates for women who are "minority, single, poorly educated and participate in the Supplemental Nutrition Program for Women, Infants and Children (WIC) are breastfeeding at the lowest rates, while many of their infants have high rates of morbidity and mortality" (Finch and Daniel 2004). Young Tabitha Walrond might have tried to defy the trend of infant formula use among the indigent, but she had neither sufficient education nor knowledgeable support from family, friends, or health practitioners to enable her to succeed with breastfeeding.

To ensure successful breastfeeding, mothers need encouragement and helpful follow-up care. Just as public health efforts were made in New York City to combat atrocious infant mortality rates in the early 1900s, the same type of efforts need to be made to educate childbearing mothers about the benefits and logistics of breastfeeding. For now, the excellent resources available to support breastfeeding mothers are geared toward women who can afford to pay for them.

In order to make breastfeeding more accessible to the general public, some Web sites on the Internet offer helpful and free educational information about breastfeeding. Dr. Jack Newman's Web site offers articles about breastfeeding, as do La Leche League, an international breastfeeding Web site called The World Alliance for Breastfeeding action, and many more Web sites. More than half of American households have access the Internet, so breastfeeding advocacy might grow well beyond its elemental stage on the World Wide Web. Ultimately, free and widespread access to sound and informative education is the key to assuring any woman's ability to succeed with breastfeeding.

BREASTFEEDING AND EDUCATION

Regrettably, even as efforts are made to increase public awareness of breastfeeding's benefits, it is not uncommon for the media to offer the general public distorted and biased information about breastfeeding. When new research demonstrates another aspect of breastfeeding's superiority, the media tend to mention the benefits with subdued interest or skepticism. They also tend to emphasize the supposed shortcomings of breastfeeding while simultaneously presenting the use of infant formula as a benign and healthy mode of infant feeding.

Simply put, the media are not averse to drawing negative attention toward breastfeeding. For example, the media widely publicized the diagnosis of Insufficient Milk Syndrome several years ago. In the mid-1990s, the *Wall Street Journal* cited an increased incidence of breastfeeding problems among middle-class suburban women. Around the same time, the television program *20/20* aired a decidedly anti-breastfeeding segment that featured a one-year-old baby who was brain-damaged as a result of experiencing dehydration as a breastfed infant. The tremendous publicity given this diagnosis promoted a long-standing myth that breastfeeding is a deficient and inferior mode of infant feeding. Concomitantly, the media communicated the overt message that infant formula is a reliable and trustworthy mode of infant feeding.

The media chose to denounce breastfeeding instead of investigating the problems that lead women to experience difficulty with breastfeeding. The fact is that most women are rarely exposed to successful breastfeeding, and breastfeeding education is frequently inadequate. The problem with breastfeeding education was stated clearly by the World Health Organization (WHO) in 1994:

> In the past two decades, there has been a rapid increase in our understanding, not only of the scientific basis of lactation and suckling, but also of effective management and prevention of breast-feeding problems, including the use of basic counselling skills. Research has shown that if health workers' attitudes and practices are supportive, it is more likely that mothers will breastfeed successfully and for a longer period. Unfortunately, breastfeeding has been neglected in the training of most health workers, leaving a serious gap in both their knowledge and skills. Training is urgently needed at all levels in up-to-date and effective breastfeeding management (WHO 2002).

The indisputable conclusion is that health care workers at all levels need to become better educated about breastfeeding if they are to help women to breastfeed successfully.

One of the main impediments to improving the education of health workers, however, is the commonly held and misguided belief that breastfeeding is instinctive. On the contrary, it is impossible for breastfeeding to be an instinct because an instinct cannot be thwarted by conscious will. Millions of women can choose not to breastfeed because they are not programmed by instinct to breastfeed.

At the same time, numerous women who wish to breastfeed may experience difficulties because they need to learn how to breastfeed. As health practitioners face the task of assisting women who have difficulty breastfeeding, they must be able to provide proper education about breastfeeding. In a way, though, it might be easier for health workers to trust that women must possess an instinct to breastfeed. In this way, they do not need to investigate to learn why women have problems with breastfeeding, and they do not need to offer help or solutions. Undoubtedly, many health practitioners feel uncomfortable broaching the subject of breastfeeding simply because breastfeeding is an intimate and private activity whereas bottle-feeding is much more impersonal and overtly acceptable.

In general, Americans are less intimate than Europeans and South Americans who generally greet one another with a hug and one, two, or even three kisses to the cheeks. Americans tend to greet one another from a distance with a wave of a hand, and this tendency is reflected in the uneasiness many people demonstrate toward breastfeeding. Thus, it is unsurprising that American health workers might be reluctant to offer advice on breastfeeding. It is, after all, easier to think that a mother who has problems with breastfeeding will eventually get the hang of it. Ultimately, adequately trained and educated health workers are needed to help mothers succeed with breastfeeding.

The World Health Organization (WHO) and United Nations Children's Fund (UNICEF) published a joint statement in 1989 entitled "Protecting, promoting and supporting breastfeeding: the special role of maternity services." They cited 10 steps that maternity services should follow to establish successful breastfeeding:

1. Have a written breastfeeding policy that is routinely communicated to all health care staff.

2. Train all health care staff in skills necessary to implement this policy.

3. Inform all pregnant women about the benefits and management of breastfeeding.

4. Help mothers initiate breastfeeding within a half hour of birth.

5. Show mothers how to breastfeed and how to maintain lactation even if they should be separated from their infants.

6. Give newborn infants no food or drink other than breast milk, unless medically indicated.

7. Practice rooming-in—allow mothers and infants to remain together—24 hours.

8. Encourage breastfeeding on demand.

9. Give no artificial teats or pacifiers (also called dummies or soothers) to breastfeeding infants.

10. Foster the establishment of breastfeeding support groups and refer mothers to them on discharge from the hospital or clinic (Lawrence 1995, 6).

The use of these detailed guidelines would help to ensure the initiation of breastfeeding and assist breastfeeding mothers once they leave the hospital. Programs like this would also help women who need assistance but cannot afford to hire a lactation consultant. By emphasizing the importance of the breastfeeding dyad as soon as possible after giving birth, the breastfeeding relationship will be that much more protected. The best way to prevent breastfeeding failure is to offer comprehensive breastfeeding education before hospital discharge and provide excellent follow-up care after hospital discharge.

In the long run, the most important way to ensure the production of abundant milk is to breastfeed a young infant around the clock. Newborns should not be sleeping through the night, and nursing every three to four hours is often insufficient to stimulate adequate milk production. A baby should be offered the breast as frequently as possible, perhaps every one to three hours in the newborn period. It is the rare mother who breastfeeds around the clock and cannot produce sufficient breast milk for her infant.

INSUFFICIENT MILK SYNDROME

Insufficient Milk Syndrome has diverse causes, and it affects less than one percent of breastfeeding mothers although a few pediatricians cite a much higher figure of up to five percent. Insufficient Milk Syndrome has been associated with varying situations. Surgical procedures such as breast reduction or breast augmentation often interfere with the normal anatomy of breast tissue. A history of sexual abuse may leave women psychologically and emotionally traumatized, such that they are unable to tolerate the physical intimacy of breastfeeding on demand. Cesarean section births may lead to breastfeeding difficulties, mainly as a result of a newborn's prolonged separation from his mother and the mother's post-surgical discomfort. The use of pain narcotics, which 50 percent of women request and receive during labor, may be transmitted to the newborn via the placenta, possibly impairing the newborn's ability to suckle and stay alert. There are also unusual circumstances, such as a possible correlation with a rare disease called Polycystic Ovary Syndrome (Marasco, Marmet, and Shell 2000).

The diagnosis of Insufficient Milk Syndrome has gained more prominence in recent years, but the information provided by the media may not necessarily be accurate. A 1999 *Newsweek* magazine article by Susan Greenberg listed the following factors that might indicate a low breast milk supply: (1) minimal or no breast changes during pregnancy; (2) lack of engorgement after delivery; (3) milk doesn't come in by fifth day; (4) no audible gulps from the baby; (5) the newborn loses more than 10 percent of his birth weight; (6) the baby produces fewer than six wet diapers daily after day three; (7) the baby produces fewer than three or four stools daily after day four; and (8) the baby seems to be nursing continuously and is never satisfied. This comprehensive and intimidating list was published in a nationally distributed newsmagazine, and it states that these factors might indicate insufficient milk production. It is not, however, entirely accurate.

Some women, for instance, do not experience breast changes during pregnancy. Pediatrician Dr. Jack Newman (2000, 30) writes that some breastfeeding mothers to not feel full breasts even though they are producing sufficient milk, especially early in the newborn period. Many breastfeeding mothers need to breastfeed on demand frequently in order to establish a bountiful supply of milk, and then they might feel full breasts. Also, it is true that the sound of a baby swallowing while suckling can be a sign of sufficient breast milk ingestion, but babies sometimes swallow silently.

The article also notes that a mother's milk should come in by the fifth day even though colostrum is normally produced for the first week, during which time the newborn has very low caloric needs. Transitional milk is produced after colostrum, and most babies do not drink mature breast milk until about two weeks after birth. The progression of breast milk maturation corresponds accurately to the nursling's physiological and nutritional needs as long as suckling is encouraged. Unfortunately, since many parents are accustomed to the less frequent but large servings of infant formula that young babies are fed, they are often unaware of how frequently a baby should be nursed at the breast.

Failure to suckle at the breast on demand and a baby's inability to latch on to the breast correctly are the primary reasons for insufficient milk production. Milk production may be impaired if breasts are not stimulated with frequent and correct suckling. Additionally, matters may be worsened when women perceive that they do not have sufficient breast milk, and they take measures that further impede success with breastfeeding.

When insufficient milk production is suspected, women are often advised to pump their breasts to quantify milk output. This action, however, may lead to a greater decline in breast milk production. Additionally, pumping may be a poor measure of breast milk production. Although electric breast pumps are good tools, they are not completely efficient tools. It is suckling at the breast that will encourage the adequate production of breast milk and the emptying of breasts.

Women who think that they do not have enough breast milk tend to supplement breastfeeding with infant formula or glucose water. While it may appear to be wise to offer a supplement when a breastfed baby does not seem to be getting enough breast milk, the introduction of a supplement often interferes significantly with the suckling that optimally stimulates adequate milk production. This interference often initiates or causes a further decline in the production of sufficient breast milk.

Lactation consultants counsel women who have difficulty breastfeeding, and the consensus appears to be that women give up easily on breastfeeding. Maria Parlapiano, director of the Lactation Resource Center in Chatham, N.J., said, "'I just didn't have enough milk' has been the No. 1 excuse for stopping breast-feeding...But often it's just a misinterpretation of the baby's behavior, like feeding every two hours" (Greenberg 1999). If women are inclined to think that infant formula is a good substitute, then insufficient milk often becomes an acceptable reason to stop breastfeeding.

It is imperative, however, for concerted efforts to be made to disseminate sound and helpful information about breastfeeding. Breastfeeding is a holistic life activity that gives young children far more than incredible breast milk. Society needs to learn once again what women throughout the history of humankind have known: breastfeeding is a source of life nourishment, and it is not an instinctive behavior that any woman manifests without effort. It takes determination and perseverance to breastfeed. Within the activity of breastfeeding, however, lies all that parents need to parent humanely and compassionately.

8

BREASTFEEDING MYTHS

Breastfeeding myths have abounded for a long time, and these unfortunate myths must be dispelled. By addressing mistaken myths about breastfeeding, it might be possible to better appreciate breastfeeding for the deeply humanizing life activity that it is. The following section is not a comprehensive analysis of either breastfeeding's negative or positive attributes. Instead, it is a brief discussion of some of the myths that lead the general public to misconstrue the importance of breastfeeding.

As mentioned earlier, breastfeeding is not a panacea. In fact, there are some contraindications to breastfeeding, which are discussed in Appendix C. Breastfeeding cannot accomplish many things, including the following: cure young children of their congenital defects or genetic deficiencies; prevent children from being exposed to infectious illnesses; guarantee that children will not be afflicted with cancer, chronic disease, or other debilitating illnesses; alter a young child's genetic make-up so that coveted genius and talent will be expressed when such genetic potential does not exist; and deter young children from experiencing unfortunate trauma or accidents in the future.

In summary, breastfeeding is not a magical solution to all of life's problems. Nevertheless, breastfeeding can provide young children the best beginning in life, however bad or good any child's life circumstances may be.

MYTH #1: BREASTFEEDING IS TOO DIFFICULT

Breastfeeding is an art that is challenging to learn in the modern era because most women are hardly exposed to breastfeeding. Women may look around in any public arena, and they will be a hundred times more likely to see a baby being fed from a bottle than from a breast. Babyhood, in many ways, is now symbolized by the ubiquitous baby bottle.

Baby births are routinely acknowledged with announcement cards that are adorned with baby bottles; baby bottles and pacifiers can be seen in the mouths of far too many babies and toddlers; nearly all grocery stores are well stocked with infant formula products and bottles; and television commercials and magazine advertisements praise the beauty of bottle-fed babies and their bottle-wielding mothers. It would not be inaccurate to note that modern culture practically excludes breastfeeding from daily life.

This does not mean, however, that the act of breastfeeding itself is difficult. Breastfeeding is a remarkably straightforward and efficient means of nourishing young children. Once women learn even a bit about the art of breastfeeding, most find out how simple it is. It appears, though, that the greatest hurdle to breastfeeding is to begin breastfeeding in the first place and then to continue for more than a few weeks.

Obstacles to initiating breastfeeding begin after childbirth and in the hospital. Unbeknownst to most women who give birth in hospitals, newborn nursery personnel have long been unpaid infant formula spokespersons. For many decades, hospital nurses have been placating crying newborns with glucose water or infant formula, both of which are produced and processed by infant formula manufacturers. If mothers insist that their babies only breastfeed, they may encounter resistant nurses who may label them as being too demanding.

I was surprised to learn that a friend of mine had such an encounter a couple of years ago in New York City. The nurses were annoyed that my friend insisted that her son not be given any infant formula or glucose water. It appears, amazingly enough, that all the gains that have been made in breast milk research have not necessarily brought about positive changes in the way hospital staff approach mothers who choose to breastfeed.

Then again, it may be difficult to discern the insidious nature of the tactics used by the infant formula industry to sell infant formula. For instance, as a practicing pediatrician I received complimentary diaper bags to distribute to my patients. At the time, I thought the bags were a nice gift to new parents even though the infant formula logo was displayed prominently on the bag. It did not occur to me that I was promoting this particular brand of infant formula.

It takes courage for parents to withstand the endless propaganda that promotes the use of infant formula. It takes fortitude for women to persevere with breastfeeding in the face of an influential infant formula industry that promotes its products irrespective of the harm it does to both babies and their mothers.

MYTH #2: BREASTFEEDING IS ONLY FOR YOUNG BABIES

There are many individuals, including physicians, who opine that breastfeeding is only for young babies. One should question, though, how it is possible to think that a growing and developing infant will thrive better on processed baby food and artificial milk substitutes than on breastfeeding. Breast milk is a living fluid that contains custom made antibodies and a perfect assortment of nutrients, live cells, immunologically active substances, growth factors, and much more. Breast milk is a dynamic substance that is manufactured in response to the needs of a growing and developing baby and toddler.

With the availability of irrefutable evidence that demonstrates the benefits of breast milk, it should be simple to defy the preconceived notion that breast milk becomes a useless fluid once the baby turns six months, one year, or even five years old. Breast milk transmits directly to nurslings the beneficial substances that complement ideally their healthy growth and development. Simply stated, there is no available food that could possibly be more nourishing for babies and young children than mother's milk.

Any food, be it processed cereal, mashed fresh organic fruit, strained vegetables, or artificial milk, cannot compare in any way to the benefits offered by breast milk. Breast milk contains a rich balance of over 200 substances, most of which can never be replicated. These substances support perfectly the rapid human brain growth that occurs in early childhood: brain volume more than doubles in the first year of life and nearly triples by the time a child is three years old (Montagu 1986, 55). In light of the tremendous brain growth and development that occurs within the first three years of life, it is mistaken to assume that older infants and toddlers do not need breast milk.

Until recently, breastfeeding was thought to have been useful until a baby was about six months old, at which time most babies experience the eruption of their first milk teeth. The presence of milk teeth, however, should not interfere with breastfeeding. If a baby bites down on the breast, it is highly likely that the baby has learned to bite down because he was given either a bottle or pacifier. An exclusively breastfed baby, however, has no need to bite down on the breast. If he does bite, a mother's response is often startling enough to discourage him from biting down again in the near future. Exclusively breastfed babies who have new milk teeth can continue to breastfeed, as can older toddlers who have twenty milk teeth.

A young child's need to breastfeed beyond six months cannot be dismissed because outdated and misinformed ideas about breastfeeding continue to be espoused. Any argument that denies the benefits of breastfeeding beyond six months has been refuted by scientists, anthropologists, and many mothers who know better. As wonderful as it is for a mother to breastfeed for six months, it would benefit everyone if babies could breastfeed for far longer. Young children should be offered the breast for as long as they wish.

MYTH #3: BABIES KNOW WHEN TO WEAN

Several women have told me that their young babies lost interest in breastfeeding, so they stopped breastfeeding. It is intriguing to hear mothers say that it is the babies who no longer wanted to breastfeed. After all, does a baby know what he wants? In reality, a baby does not know at all what he wants although he knows what he needs.

If a mother does not offer the breast on demand when the baby needs to nurse, he will learn as a matter of course that the breast is not a reliable presence in his life. From early on, he may learn that the breast cannot be depended upon and that he can do without it. Even though he still needs to breastfeed, the frustration of not getting breastfed often enough might lead him to eventually refuse the breast.

It is parents who teach young babies that they do not want to breastfeed since young babies are incapable of deciding for themselves how they will fulfill their needs. All babies know is that they need to cooperate with their caregivers in order to survive. Thus, if a mother does not wish to breastfeed, then the baby can protest but not for long; he will acclimate himself to the absence of the breast.

Ideally, parents should understand better the benefits of prolonged breastfeeding, and they should permit a child to determine when he is ready to stop breastfeeding. For instance, I have a friend in Ohio whose twin toddlers determined when they would stop breastfeeding. Around the time the twins had cut back to occasional breastfeeding, my friend attended a three-day conference in California. Much to her surprise, she learned that even sporadic breastfeeding may lead to copious milk production. On her first evening away from her twins, she had to buy a manual breast pump in order to relieve her engorged breasts.

A few days later, on the way home from the airport, my friend and her family were stranded on the side of the road with a flat tire. While her husband fixed the flat tire, the cranky and tired twins decided to start nursing. The children were comforted greatly by breastfeeding, and they wound up nursing regularly until they decided to stop a couple of months later. The twins' decision to stop breastfeeding is a good example of child-led weaning. In a sense, both children were old enough to comprehend the meaning of choosing to stop breastfeeding.

MYTH #4: BREASTFEEDING ON DEMAND SPOILS CHILDREN

Women have been warned for decades that they will spoil their children if they respond too readily to their children's needs. Mothers are supposed to treat babies and children with restraint and keep them at a distance. Child-rearing experts admonish repeatedly that babies should not fall asleep at the breast. These experts decry the possibility that a baby might become too dependent upon the breast and the mother.

Child-rearing experts advise instead that a young baby should learn how to comfort himself with an inanimate object and certainly not a living object like a breast. Suitable inanimate objects include a blanket, safe baby toys, a pacifier, or even a mother's shirt. In this way, the baby will learn that he is alone in this world and surrounded by inert objects that comfort him while his mother stays away to suppress her maternal urges.

I have a friend who relayed how difficult it was to rear her young children in the mid-1960s. The subject of breastfeeding did not even arise since feeding with infant formula was the norm. What pained my friend were the edicts of the pediatrician who told her how to rear her children. She was not to spoil her children by comforting them with her love and warm embrace. She was to keep her distance and keep in check her silly maternal emotions.

Mothers who distance themselves purposefully from their young children suppress maternal intuition and unknowingly punish their children. Young children need warm and loving human interaction, and nowhere is such affection displayed more clearly than when mothers breastfeed young children on demand. Breastfeeding on demand bestows upon young children the security of knowing that they are cared for and loved. Breastfeeding on demand helps to rear healthy young children who understand the meaning of love since the offering of breastfeeding on demand is an act of love.

Ashley Montagu wrote often that children are not spoiled by receiving love but by not receiving love. This is an important perspective since it defies the common understanding of what spoils children. It is the absence of love that leads children to become spoiled whereas children who are loved adequately will learn how to live as healthy and caring individuals. Thus, children who tend to demonstrate spoiled behavior did not receive sufficient love in early childhood; hence, they crave attention and affection.

Sadly and ironically, many children may experience deprivation of love and maternal affection as a result of parents' persistent effort to purportedly prevent their children from becoming spoiled. Although women throughout human history undertook breastfeeding as a nurturing and loving expression of maternal concern, only a minority of women hold such a view today. What is more commonly accepted in today's child-rearing practices is the withholding of love and the denial of breastfeeding's importance. Such deprivation, however, has fueled the widespread need for many individuals to search to find the love and security that they should have experienced during early childhood.

Individuals with good family relations and friendships may have the opportunity to speak and share with others their concerns about life. In the modern era, however, many individuals are too busy to take the time to listen to one another. Consequently, there has been a long-standing and ever-increasing demand for therapists and analysts. For those children and adults who can afford the therapy, there may be hope that they can learn how to rectify whatever troubles them about their existence, including perhaps the inability to love and to be loved.

The British psychiatrist Anthony Storr (1988, 7) offers the following intriguing perspective on the analytical encounter: "In no other situation in life can anyone count on a devoted listener who is prepared to give so much time and skilled attention to the problems of a single individual without asking for any reciprocal return, other than professional remuneration. The patient may never have encountered anyone in his life who has paid him such attention or even been prepared to listen to his problems."

Storr's assessment of the unique role of a skilled analyst seems to deny the importance of the mother-child relationship. His perspective, however, makes sense since the value of mothering has become so demeaned over the past few decades. In a world that esteems mothering, nevertheless, Storr's description of a skilled analyst would fit to a tee all loving and attentive mothers.

The majority of mothers are devoted, reliable, attentive, interested, and available; they also do not expect remuneration. In addition, breastfeeding mothers are physically more available for their young children, offer profound nurturing at the breast, and are generally highly attuned to their nurslings' needs. Undoubtedly, loving and attentive breastfeeding mothers provide even greater attention than the most skilled analyst could possibly offer. It is perhaps exactly this type of attention early in life that would diminish the need for therapy and analysis later in life.

As more parents comprehend the value of breastfeeding as a humane parenting tool, the above statement could be revised so that the first sentence will begin as follows: "In no other situation in life, other than the breastfeeding dyad between mother and infant or mother and toddler, can anyone count on a devoted listener…" Ultimately, it is much easier, less expensive, and more enjoyable to learn the meaning of love at the breast than it is to learn the same lesson on a therapist's couch. In the final analysis, it is sufficient love that permits children to avoid becoming spoiled.

Some may argue that this analogy is faulty since little verbal communication occurs between a breastfeeding mother and her baby. This may be true, but one has to consider how much more difficult it is to communicate in the absence of speech. The fact that mothers take the time and make the effort to understand their babies is of supreme importance in helping young children to eventually learn how to articulate their concerns and problems to others. An individual who is able to express concerns accurately and meaningfully does not exhibit spoiled behavior.

Many children are now growing up, however, without the consistent presence and availability of a maternal figure. These children may not be able to easily articulate their angst. Frustrated and miserable, these children may exhibit the spoiled behavior that so repels many parents. The development of such behavior could be prevented, however, if more children received the intimacy of loving and attentive maternal care.

MYTH #5: BREASTFEEDING IS OPTIONAL

Breastfeeding is not always possible since families may face unforeseen circumstances such as serious maternal illness, unexpected maternal death, parental abandonment, extreme poverty or misfortune that precludes the possibility of breastfeeding, and other unusual situations. Additionally, there will always be a minority of women who will not breastfeed for varying reasons. In other words, there will be situations in which it may be difficult or perhaps impossible for women to breastfeed their babies.

Prior to the twentieth century, it was inconceivable that breastfeeding would be treated as an optional mode of infant feeding. Breastfeeding was widely recognized as being critical to infant survival. This mind-set changed significantly with the advent of improved water sanitation, pasteurization of animal milk, and the commercial production of infant formula. As it became evident that more infants were able to survive without breastfeeding, the proposition that a select minority of infants could benefit from artificial milk feedings gradually gave way to the commonly held supposition that healthy infants could thrive in the absence of breastfeeding. Hence, the current and popular view of breastfeeding is that it is optional.

More and more, breastfeeding is viewed to be not only optional but also completely expendable. Historian Marilyn Yalom (1997, 239) offers the following bizarre conclusion about infant feeding in *A History of the Breast*: "We now know why breast milk is beneficial to infants: the hormones and enzymes that promote growth and the antibodies that protect against common infections have been largely identified. Those who choose not to breast-feed no longer need worry about the health of bottle-fed babies, if the formula is properly prepared and administered." The first sentence is accurate although there are still substances in breast milk that have not yet been identified or whose roles have not yet been fully clarified. The second sentence, though, is egregiously wrong because infant formula does not at all contain the hormones, enzymes, and antibodies that are found in breast milk.

Simply because these active substances have been identified in breast milk does not mean, in any way, that they all now exist in infant formula. As mentioned earlier, infant formula manufacturers know that it is impossible to replicate breast milk, and they do not even attempt to do so. This is why infant formula contains a paltry minimum of 29 ingredients versus more than 200 ingredients that are found naturally in breast milk. Even so, Yalom can write without compunction that parents "no longer need worry about the health of bottle-fed babies."

It would be wonderful if there was no need to worry about the health of infant formula-fed babies, but young babies and children have health problems, and they can no longer be ignored. For example, over 15 percent of children between the ages of six and nineteen are obese, and there have been significant increases in the prevalence of overweight and obese children under the age of five years. An American Academy of Pediatrics Policy Statement noted that obese children are at risk for developing elevated cholesterol and lipids, high blood pressure, Type 2 diabetes mellitus, impaired glucose tolerance, insulin resistance, menstrual irregularities, depression, and low self-esteem (AAP 2003).

These significant obesity-related health hazards should not be experienced by so many children, and fewer children would be overweight or obese if they were breastfed. Breastfeeding, as the same AAP policy statement noted, decreases the risk of obesity later in life: "Extent and duration of breastfeeding have been found to be inversely associated with risk of obesity in later childhood, possibly mediated by physiologic factors in human milk as well as by the feeding and parenting patterns associated with nursing." Thus, the longer a child breastfeeds, the lower is his risk of becoming obese later in life.

A recent study published in *Circulation,* a medical journal of the American Heart Association, determined that formula-fed babies who gained weight rapidly during the first week of life were significantly more likely to be overweight or obese decades later (Stettler et al. 2005). The study recommends that babies be breastfed.

As discussed earlier, breastfeeding is increasingly being recognized for its unique capabilities in fending off or mitigating infectious illnesses. This is significant since bottle-fed children are at higher risk of becoming ill with acute and chronic infections. Over the past two to three decades, the excessive use of antibiotics in the pediatric population has played an important role in the emergence of bacteria that are resistant to many commonly used antibiotics. There is genuine concern that antibiotics one day will be ineffective in treating serious bacterial infections in children and adults alike.

In *Breaking the Antibiotic Habit,* infectious disease specialist Dr. Paul A. Offit and his colleagues offer guidelines that would decrease the incidence of antibiotic use for various children's illnesses. They offer this gloomy assessment of antibiotic use in the introduction to their book: "The reason that some bacteria have become resistant to antibiotics is that antibiotics are *overused.* Children are the most common victims of this overuse. Of the roughly 145 million antibiotic prescriptions written every year, most are written for young children. The result is that young children are more likely to be infected by highly resistant bacteria than any other group" (Offit, Offit, and Bell 1999, 1). Their legitimate concern is that the use of antibiotics as a treatment against infection may soon be ineffective and that children may suffer inordinately as a result of prevalent antibiotic prescribing practices.

Although the primary medical approach to treating illness is to find and use the appropriate medication or therapy, it is probably even more important to try to prevent the occurrence of illness in the first place. Hence, breastfeeding's significance as a preventive health tool is immeasurable since research continues to elucidate the many benefits that breastfeeding passes on to nurslings. Breastfeeding provides both active and passive immunity. It is not an exaggeration to write that breastfeeding is probably the most effective and beneficial preventive measure available to ensure good long-term health for human beings.

As important as preventive measures like breastfeeding may be, the maintenance of good health is predicated upon future health habits. Consequently, a breastfed baby who winds up smoking three packs of cigarettes a day as an adult will injure his lungs and heart. Similarly, a breastfed baby who is subsequently fed a regular diet of copious amounts of fast food will invariably become overweight or obese. Environmental factors influence the health of all individuals, including those who are breastfed as babies. Since breastfeeding is not a panacea, breastfed babies may develop infectious illnesses, acute illnesses, chronic diseases, or cancer.

The breastfed baby who does experience illness, however, receives unsurpassable nourishment and numerous active substances to either fight off or ameliorate the severity of the afflicting disease. For the most part, breastfed babies experience disease or infection differently from those who are bottle-fed with infant formula. For example, a baby or toddler who has fever, vomiting, or diarrhea needs nourishment and hydration. Sick babies and young children often lose their appetites and can hardly tolerate ingesting most foods and liquids, including infant formula. Breast milk, however, is an ideal source of oral replenishment for babies and young toddlers since it contains nearly 90 percent water and a perfect complement of electrolytes. Breastfed children also enjoy the comfort and nourishment of breast milk when they are ill.

Moreover, breastfed babies receive important psychological and emotional succor from breastfeeding. When babies experience pain or suffering, breastfeeding provides intimacy and comfort. Consequently, breastfed children who are ill are often able to sleep through the night. Whether it is the comfort and assurance provided by the breast or the drowsing effect of breast milk, the benefit of getting a sick baby or child to sleep is enormous.

Breastfeeding is much more than a choice of infant feeding, and it is surely not optional. Breastfeeding can be a primary tool to support the health and well-being of young babies and children. With better education, it is possible that breastfeeding can become a part of a healthier way of life for many more Americans.

MYTH #6: BREASTFEEDING IS INCONVENIENT

Despite the greater convenience of breastfeeding, it is popularly believed that the use of infant formula is convenient. In reality, bottle-feeding is both time-consuming and preoccupying. Parents have to remember to bring along infant formula wherever they go, particularly during the first six months of life when a baby only breastfeeds or drinks formula. If parents unintentionally run out of infant formula, they will discover that they cannot purchase infant formula anywhere, at any time, and for a reasonable price.

In comparison, nearly everything about breastfeeding revolves around convenience. Breast milk is produced on demand at the perfect temperature and in idealized quantities. A breastfeeding mother needs only to perhaps lift a shirt or unclasp a nursing bra. Otherwise, breastfeeding is completely ready and available to fulfill a baby's needs.

As a rule, a nursing mother should try to keep herself hydrated with water and nourished with well balanced meals. Amazingly, even when a nursing mother is not well nourished, the breastfed baby can still extract sustenance that complements his good health. Uncluttered by miscellaneous paraphernalia such as bottles, infant formula, water, and rubber nipples, a mother can breastfeed nearly any place and at any time.

For example, several years ago a young couple, Jim and Jennifer Stolpa, and their infant son, Clayton, were stranded in a blizzard in Nevada for over a week. The mother kept herself hydrated by ingesting snow, and she supplemented the baby's breastfeeding with snow she melted in her mouth. The breastfed five-month-old baby survived in excellent condition even though his mother had run out of food several days earlier.

Breastfeeding is both possible and beneficial under less than ideal circumstances. If the baby had been bottle-fed and infant formula was unavailable, the baby might have suffered a far different fate. Breastfeeding is truly far more convenient and life-saving than is generally acknowledged.

MYTH #7: BREASTFEEDING IS DANGEROUS

Recently, concerns have been raised about toxins that may be transmitted through breast milk to nurslings. Such research is legitimate since the human environment is most certainly contaminated with man-made substances. Unfortunately, we now live in an era that is highly dependent upon technology, and various dangerous chemicals and toxic substances are used to manufacture many goods that are omnipresent in the home, at work, and in the community.

Increasingly, human beings are exposed to substances that were unheard of a century ago, such as the following: banned pesticides like DDT, banned industrial chemicals like flame retardants (PBDEs, for example), and banned coolants like PCBs. These types of substances are particularly harmful because they persist in the environment and perhaps in the human body. Some of these substances are fat-soluble and, thus, may persist in the fat tissue of the human body. They will be present in higher concentrations in women since women have a higher percentage of fat in their bodies than do men. Consequently, breast milk may contain some of these fat soluble toxins.

The question of whether or not breast milk is "toxic" is not viewed, however, with an appreciation for the overall benefits breastfeeding may bestow upon both children and mothers. Breastfeeding is seen, instead, from the perspective of its expendability: it is automatically assumed that breastfeeding is unnecessary if there is a remote possibility of its being "harmful." This is the case since the culture of bottle-feeding with infant formula prevails in the Western world. In light of the toxins that may be present in breast milk, it is feared that breastfeeding may poison a baby or child.

Meanwhile, the gold standard of safety is assumed to be infant formula even though, as mentioned earlier, infant formula may be contaminated by bacteria, and it supplies less than 40 ingredients compared to over 200 naturally occurring substances in breast milk. The sources of milk used to manufacture infant formula, as discussed earlier, may be laced with pesticides, fungicides, antibiotics, and other substances, but there are no media reports of investigations to determine what types of toxins are found in infant formula. This makes no sense since the toxins that have been found in women's breast milk are present primarily in the environment, including the water that is used to process infant formula in factories and reconstitute powdered or dilute concentrated liquid infant formula in the home.

The cavalier way in which breast milk is treated as a mere mode of infant feeding ignores the entire process of breastfeeding. Breastfeeding is not just a source of breast milk: it is a complicated and intricate physiological process that produces a highly purified and complex liquid. Numerous control mechanisms on the cellular level are involved in the accurate production of breast milk that best nourishes the breastfeeding baby. The homeostatic concentrations of electrolytes and minerals in breast milk, for example, are not created by chance. There are feedback mechanisms that control precisely what goes into the production of human milk.

Breastfeeding is a dynamic and responsive physiological process. Although it is highly disturbing that the environment of the average American citizen is polluted enough that toxins are found in breast milk, it appears that a breastfeeding mother's body is capable of responding to the undesirable presence of such poisonous substances. In other words, the composition of breast milk may be adjusted in order to perhaps counter or mitigate the effects of such toxins on the nursing baby or child.

In an article entitled "Toxic Breast Milk?" in the January 9, 2005, issue of the *New York Times Magazine*, Florence Williams reports that studies have been done to determine the effects of PCBs on children. PCBs are considered to be harmful and a probable carcinogen. Williams cites research that was performed in the Great Lakes region, the Arctic, and the Netherlands. She writes that "babies born to mothers with mid-to upper-range background levels of PCB contamination (probably because of diets rich in contaminated fish and animal products), have delayed learning capabilities, lower I.Q.'s, and reduced immunities against infections." The studies showed that children who were breastfed had higher levels of PCBs as compared to children who were exposed to PCBs in the womb and were not breastfed.

Intriguingly, the conclusion of these studies does not lead to a condemnation of breastfeeding. Even though the breastfed children had higher levels of PCBs, these children "consistently performed better than those who drank formula." Unsurprising to those who understand that breastfeeding is a complex process that specifically protects nurslings, it appears that breast milk may offer some protection against the effects of toxic substances in breast milk. Thus, the World Health Organization (WHO) and other groups recommend that women continue to breastfeed.

As human beings continue to pollute the environment, more human beings may be exposed to the toxic effects of unnatural and harmful substances. The only way to prevent such risks is to stop the creation and use of pollutants. Historically, when sufficient scientific information determines that specific chemicals are toxic or the public demands accountability from the U.S. government, the specific substances may be banned. Unfortunately, the chemicals may linger in the environment for decades, during which time human beings will continue to be exposed to the toxins.

An infant who grows and develops in a polluted environment needs protection from pollutants. Parents can do their best to avoid exposing their infants and toddlers to harmful chemicals. Parents can also use breastfeeding, which is a unique filtering system within nursing women's bodies, to produce ideal nourishment and numerous protective substances that complement a baby's growing and developing body.

MYTH #8: BREASTFEEDING AND HIV

The American Academy of Pediatrics advises women in the U.S. who are infected with HIV not to breastfeed. This is undoubtedly the case since there is a real risk of transmitting HIV through breastfeeding. More research needs to be done, however, in order to clarify the true risk of transmitting HIV through breastfeeding and the ways in which such HIV transmission may be prevented (by treating mother and baby with anti-viral medications, perhaps).

In developing countries, non-breastfed babies may face a greater risk of illness or death as a result of contracting infections other than HIV infection. This is particularly true for women who face poverty and poor water sanitation. In such situations, women probably cannot afford infant formula, and water is generally not sanitary enough to avoid infection with parasites, bacteria, and viruses.

There are millions of women with HIV infection in poorer countries, and continued research is being done to clarify in which situations breastfeeding in the presence of HIV infection might be possible or beneficial. Such research will eventually assist women who are infected with HIV but wish to breastfeed their babies.

Anna Coutsoudis offered an update on current research related to HIV infection and breastfeeding in the February 2005 issue of *Breastfeeding Abstracts.* Current evidence demonstrates a 0.74% risk of HIV transmission to a nursling for every month the baby is breastfed (Coutsoudis 2005). This means that a baby who is breastfed for six months may experience a 4% risk of becoming infected with HIV: this is a risk few parents in the Western world would tolerate.

Recent research demonstrates, however, that a woman who is infected with HIV may breastfeed without increasing the risk of transmitting the virus to her nursling. One prospective study from South Africa determined that the cumulative risk of HIV infection for exclusively breastfed infants who drank only breast milk for the first six months of life was the same as if the baby was not breastfed at all (Coutsoudis 2005). The risk of transmission was increased, however, when babies received a mixture of both breastfeeding and bottle-feeding with infant formula. Other studies performed in Africa confirmed the finding that exclusively breastfed babies had a lower risk of HIV infection as compared to babies who received mixed feedings with both breastfeeding and bottle-feeding.

In the U.S., the advice for women to avoid breastfeeding in the presence of HIV infection is accepted de facto. This is the case since infant formula feeding has long been a standard American child-rearing practice. Even though women all over the world throughout history have breastfed and continue to breastfeed their babies, breastfeeding in the U.S. is no longer a practice that is well understood. To many Americans, it only makes sense that HIV-infected women should not breastfeed. After all, most of the general public and the health community either do not know of or deny the serious health risks that are associated with bottle-feeding.

In the U.S., the majority of women who are infected with HIV will most likely not be bothered by the advice to avoid breastfeeding. There are other women, however, who had planned to breastfeed their babies; they will find little support for breastfeeding. Undoubtedly, in light of evidence that HIV can be transmitted through breast milk, few health practitioners would advise a woman infected with HIV to breastfeed. The majority of health practitioners do not want to be held legally responsible for giving advice that might lead to HIV transmission to nurslings. Besides, the culture of breastfeeding is not at all established in the medical community, so expert physicians would not advocate breastfeeding in the presence of HIV infection.

A small minority of women with HIV infection wish to breastfeed, and there are some women who are successfully breastfeeding their babies. For example, the August 19, 2000, issue of *Newsweek* magazine features an article by David France about Christine Maggiore, a woman in Los Angeles who is infected with HIV. At the time of the interview, she was breastfeeding her healthy three-year-old son with the support of her child's pediatrician. Maggiore is an atypical activist who believes that HIV does not cause AIDS.

Maggiore and her child's pediatrician are unusual, and perhaps reckless to those who are accustomed to thinking that the use of infant formula is benign. In the U.S., few women and pediatricians trust the importance of breastfeeding enough to defy current recommendations against breastfeeding in the presence of HIV infection. With greater research, however, it is possible that those who support breastfeeding's irreplaceable role in child-rearing will be vindicated and permitted to encourage women with HIV infection to breastfeed their babies without harming them.

For now, Dr. Jack Newman (2000, 281) describes two alternatives for women who are infected with HIV but still wish to offer their babies breast milk. He suggests either banked breast milk or expressed breast milk that is treated with heat. Banked breast milk consists of breast milk that various women have donated, and it is processed so that some immune factors are reduced or eliminated. Banked milk still offers greater nutritional value than any infant formula product. The second suggestion entails that women express breast milk and heat the milk to 140 degrees for 30 minutes, which is sufficient to kill the virus. The technology for heating the breast milk at home is imperfect, so Dr. Newman recommends that the breast milk be treated at a local hospital.

PART II

IN DEFENSE OF MOTHERING AND FAMILY LIFE

9

THE SEPARATION OF BABIES FROM MOTHERS

WHATEVER HAPPENED TO STAY-AT-HOME MOTHERING?

The widespread use of infant formula and the mass exodus of mothers of young children from the home and into the workforce are now the norm. Increasingly, parents trust that breastfeeding and the provision of hands-on maternal care are archaic and unnecessary parenting practices. This is assumed since babies and children appear to grow, develop, and survive without breastfeeding and maternal care.

Although only a minority of children might have experienced such deprivation in the past, it is now the minority of children who experience the benefits of breastfeeding and hands-on maternal care. In the past, the youngsters who had to survive in the absence of breastfeeding and maternal care were relatively anomalous. The combination of the uniqueness of their predicament and the hope for their survival was dramatic enough to become the basis of story lines for many children's books and films.

Consider, for example, the protagonists of Disney animated films like *Bambi, Snow White and the Seven Dwarves, Cinderella, The Hunchback of Notre Dame, The Little Mermaid,* and *Finding Nemo.* The leading characters all experience maternal deprivation during their youth: either their mothers are dead before the story begins (Snow White, Cinderella, and Ariel) or they are murdered soon after the story begins (Bambi, Esmeralda, and Nemo). The mothers' absence is sad and frightening, but it is also almost irrelevant because the children receive loving surrogate or paternal care.

The maturation of these characters and their ability to survive despite the hardship of not receiving maternal care attest to the resilience of human beings. The children's survival also reflects their innate potential and subsequent manifestation of their goodness and intelligence, as well as their ingenuity, adaptability, and will to survive. The basic message behind these stories is that children will survive or even thrive despite the experience of maternal deprivation.

Like these fictional film characters, the present majority of children experience maternal deprivation and are expected not only to survive but to succeed in life. The absence of hands-on mothering from current child-rearing practices occurs frequently, however, not as a result of extenuating circumstances such as death or maternal illness but as a result of parental choice. The vast majority of young babies and children today have mothers, but many women simply no longer take care of their own children.

Contrary to popular belief, the transformation of maternal care from a hands-on activity to a supervisory role in modern child-rearing practices did not evolve naturally. Systematic efforts on various fronts have been made for over a century to discourage women from breastfeeding and providing maternal care. Although women cared directly for their young babies and children throughout human history, the majority of women today feel compelled to return to work outside the home and leave the care of their young babies and children to others. One should wonder how and why the modern lifestyle has changed so dramatically that it practically precludes breastfeeding and the provision of hands-on maternal care for even the youngest of babies.

Although a majority of women do initiate breastfeeding in the newborn period, the fall off is significant in early infancy. Undoubtedly, the pressure to return to work outside the home dissuades many women from continuing to breastfeed. Additionally, the infant formula industry has convinced countless parents that the use of infant formula is easier and more convenient than the bother of breastfeeding and breast pumping. In blatant defiance of biology and common sense, the prevailing attitude toward breastfeeding and hands-on maternal care is that it is irrelevant to the well-being of young babies, mothers, and family life as a whole.

This view of breastfeeding and women's work has been created and nurtured most forcefully by feminists who champion indefatigably the persistent presence of women in the workforce. Their advocacy of women's participation in the work world is admirable and imperative since women need and deserve to have the opportunity to contribute to the work world. To trust, however, that the majority of children will thrive in the absence of loving maternal care is ludicrous. This is, nevertheless, the primary assumption made by feminists as they obsess that women who stay home will set back or perhaps erase the gains made by the women's movement in the work world. Popular culture even promotes the idea that a woman's decision to stay home and leave the workforce is contrary to women's true nature.

This was unmistakably the message conveyed in the 2004 film *The Stepford Wives*, which is a remake of a 1975 film that was based upon a novel by Ira Levin. In the recent version of the film, the men of Stepford realize their conception of a perfect spouse as someone who stays home and exists to serve primarily the man's needs. The men go to extremes to control their wives (and one gay partner), forcing them to shed their natural personas, which is to be dominant, intelligent, ambitious, high-powered, and successful. According to the film, staying home to care for husband and home (as well as children, who play minor roles in the story line) is merely aberrant behavior for the modern woman.

Another view of suburban homemakers is offered on the new hit television show *Desperate Housewives*. It offers a dark and comedic view of unhappy suburban housewives from the perspective of a fellow housewife who has committed suicide. The show is a prime time soap opera that features photogenic women and their encounters with sex, deception, frustration, depression, and intrigue. In the not-so-distant future, the fictional women characters of *Desperate Housewives* will become emblematic of early twenty-first century homemakers in the same way that June Cleaver and Donna Reed symbolize 1950s housewives in popular culture today.

On a show like *Desperate Housewives*, I doubt that breastfeeding is a subject that is broached since the primary point of the show is to emphasize the drama of being unfulfilled housewives. There is little or no ado associated with women who are content with breastfeeding, child-rearing, and stay-at-home mothering. In contrast, frustrated, unhappy, and angry women provide good fodder for entertaining story lines.

Some feminists may delight in this show's existence since it highlights the aggravation and disappointment women may experience after choosing to become homemakers. For instance, one of the show's main characters, Lynette Scavo, is a high-powered executive who regrets having given up her successful career in order to care for her four unmanageable children. She is also addicted to Ritalin that has been prescribed to treat her twins for Attention Deficit Disorder. Lynette Scavo is a fictional character, but her experience as a disgruntled and overwhelmed housewife epitomizes most women's worst nightmare: no sensible and intelligent woman wishes to lose her self-identity and sense of purpose in life as does Scavo.

Contemporary women truly fear losing their self-identity. This is especially the case when sincere efforts to nurture the well-being of one's children may be thwarted by the seemingly dysfunctional nature of modern family life. *Desperate Housewives* offers the discouraging and pessimistic perspective that modern family life is in a state of serious and perhaps irreparable disarray.

The implication is that women have little control over or responsibility for the state of the modern family. It is almost as if women are merely passive observers rather than active participants in family life. In other words, family life will be what it is regardless of what sacrifices women make in order to nurture their young children to the best of their ability. One can surmise from this perspective that the modern era is not conducive for women to rear children and partake in family life.

IDEAL CHILD-REARING IN THE DISTANT PAST

Looking back in history, there was at least one specific period of time when conditions were ideal for women to rear children. That era was some nine thousand years ago in the Neolithic or New Stone Age. In his seminal book *The Natural Superiority of Women*, Ashley Montagu describes the work of Marija Gimbutas, archaeologist and professor of European archaeology at the University of California, Los Angeles.

Gimbutas studied artifacts, which were predominantly women who were depicted as being large breasted with big buttocks and hips, corpulent, pregnant, or near childbirth. Gimbutas identified these figurines to be goddesses or fertility figures. The predominance of feminine figurines and the scarcity of male figurines suggest the powerful role women played in prehistoric societies. Ashley Montagu (1999, 72) offers a clarification of Gimbutas' conclusion: "What Gimbutas is saying is not that there ever was a society governed by women, a matriarchate, but there were many societies (if not all) that were gylanic, where women and men shared an equal partnership, and that the deities these societies celebrated were predominantly feminine."

Ashley Montagu cites the example of the Minoan culture of ancient Crete to describe a gylanic society in which women played a central role in the workings of that society. Evidently, complete equality existed between men and women, and descent was tracked in the female line. For fifteen hundred years, from about 3000 B.C. to 1500 B.C., the people of Crete "pursued the even tenor of their way, without war or conflict of any kind" (1999, 73). In other words, ancient societies that deified women's childbearing and nurturing abilities were characterized by peace, cooperation, and freedom.

Modern society could learn a great deal from these prehistoric societies since the modern world is characterized not by peace and cooperation but by warfare and competition. In fact, it is highly probable that if modern culture were to appreciate women's fertility and the ability to breastfeed, then modern society would be far more peaceful. It is a pity that the modern era is so far removed from the New Stone Age, but it is encouraging to learn that there was once a time when childbearing and breastfeeding were both greatly appreciated and admired.

It is time now to create a new culture that is cognizant of the importance of both breastfeeding on demand and stay-at-home mothering. Unfortunately, child-rearing experts continue to offer parents facile views of parenting, the latest being that parental care is irrelevant to the well-being of children. There is little doubt that human ancestors of the distant past would be appalled by the callous advice that is offered to parents by modern day child-rearing experts.

MATERNAL DEPRIVATION

Judith Rich Harris, the author of *The Nurture Assumption*, made a huge impact on child-rearing philosophy several years ago. She asserts that peer influence is far more important than parental influence is to the mental and emotional development of children. Harris says that "parents, contrary to nearly a century of scientific doctrine, have no lasting effects on the personality, intelligence or mental health of their offspring" (Sleek 1998). Carrying this theory further, Harris opines that parents are not responsible for the outcome of their children's development since parents have no meaningful influence.

Harris' theory about child-rearing may be tenable if one assumes that breastfeeding is not an integral part of parental nurturing practices. When parents do not breastfeed, they do not use a consistently intimate and caring means of communicating their concern and affection to their young children. This assertion is not meant to trivialize or deny the significance of non-breastfeeding parents' efforts to offer their children the best of care. Rather, it is to elucidate how the lack of breastfeeding may result in the failure to bridge the physical and emotional distance that exists between the nurtured and their nurturers.

Fundamentally, breastfeeding offers young babies and children a significantly greater amount of physical intimacy than does bottle-feeding. Breastfed babies can touch and feel the warmth of their mothers' bodies while they simultaneously experience the pleasure and satisfaction of drinking warm and nourishing milk straight from the breast. The pleasure that babies experience at the breast is rarely discussed, but it is of immense importance to the healthy development of young children.

Research neuroscientist James Prescott worked for nearly two decades at the National Institute of Health, and his understanding of parental care differs starkly from that of Harris. Whereas Harris disregards parental care and influence, Prescott stresses the importance of early childhood nurturing and its beneficial effects upon healthy human development. Prescott posits the theory that an insufficient amount of infant nurturing via breastfeeding, touch, warm and affectionate verbal contact, and baby carrying may lead to violent adult behavior. Prescott (1975) writes, "I am now convinced that the deprivation of physical sensory pleasure is the principal root cause of violence."

Prescott's observations are cogent since increasing numbers of children are being denied the nurturing of prolonged breastfeeding and loving hands-on maternal care. If current child-rearing trends persist, the majority of babies and children will experience the type of sensory deprivation that Prescott asserts will affect human behavior adversely. Although sensory deprivation has always existed to some degree in most populations throughout history, it is pervasive in the U.S. since the majority of babies and children today are bottle-fed and receive non-maternal care.

Some will argue that adults today are the products of 1950s child-rearing practices that included sensory deprivation in the form of detached parenting from depressed mothers and absent fathers, as well as bottle-feeding with infant formula. For some reason, this is supposed to be reassuring. The fact that many adults today survived poor parenting reflects the resilience of human beings and little more than that. The perverse assumption, however, seems to be that if adults were able to survive less than ideal child-rearing practices in the past, then their children should be able to display similar resilience in the face of even greater sensory deprivation.

Such an assumption is unfortunate since there is a huge difference in the type of sensory deprivation young babies and children experience today in comparison to what their counterparts experienced in the 1950s. Young babies and children today are deprived of both breastfeeding and maternal care. In contrast, although the majority of children might have been bottle-fed in the 1950s, most received the benefits of hands-on maternal care, irrespective of the quality of that care. Simply stated, the absence of maternal care in the modern era is a substantial difference from past child-rearing practices. Far too many young children are exposed currently to the experience of significant sensory deprivation in early childhood.

As more children experience such sensory deprivation, it is probable that the number of individuals who may not be able to overcome the experience of receiving inadequate childhood nurturing will increase. These individuals may wind up succumbing to human afflictions as varied as substance abuse, alcohol abuse, domestic abuse, mental illness, homelessness, chronic unemployment, a propensity toward committing crime and violence, and more behavior that is not well regarded by society at large.

Although human beings are resilient and they possess the potential to overcome different kinds of adversity, one cannot take for granted all children's ability to be strong and flexible enough to mature into healthy, sociable, and productive adults. Naturally, individual situations will vary and outcomes may be excellent despite bottle-feeding and the absence of maternal care. In the majority of these cases, the surrogate caregiver is a loving relative or an unusually sensitive and caring non-relative.

For example, I know a couple who reared their granddaughter since she was a newborn. At the time of the child's birth, her parents were embroiled in serious marital and financial troubles. Both parents worked long hours outside of the home, so the maternal grandparents undertook the entire responsibility of rearing the baby. She was dropped off at their house early in the morning in her pajamas, and she left late at night, bathed and dressed in clean pajamas. The grandparents oversaw the baby's care as she suffered through allergies and discomfort that arose from the use of several infant formulas. They bought the infant formula, the diapers, and they dedicated their entire lives to her well-being. Thanks to the devotion of her dedicated grandparents, the child is now a healthy and loving adolescent.

The extended family living in one house or even in the same neighborhood is most certainly no longer the norm. The availability of diverse educational and employment opportunities across the country compels many young adults to move away from their parents and their hometowns. There are, however, families who depend highly upon grandparents to offer child care services.

Timothy Williams reports in the *New York Times* on May 21, 2005, that in 2000 there were 84,000 grandparent-headed homes in New York City, as compared to 14,000 in 1991. Approximately 7 percent of American grandparents provide extensive care for their grandchildren (more than 30 hours of care per week or at least 90 nights per year), including 20 percent who provide care for pre-school aged children for parents who work outside the home (Senior Journal 2005). Increasingly, though, in the absence of an extended family structure, many babies are simply placed in the care of non-relatives such as babysitters, nannies, or day care workers.

The trend to place babies in the care of non-family caregivers or institutions is a momentous change in child-rearing that is, strangely enough, not addressed with great concern. For the greater part of human existence, maternal care was the most likely source of loving and pleasurable sensory stimulation for children's healthy growth and development. In sharp contrast, it has become fairly common for many young children to experience maternal deprivation. Whether the majority of children can handle such experiences is clearly a matter of chance.

Some families are fortunate since they are able to procure excellent and affectionate substitute care for their children. For instance, I know an adorable set of toddler twins whose mother owns a business and works out of the home frequently. For many years now, one nanny has been the consistent caregiver for the family, which includes the young twins as well as their two elder adolescent siblings.

This nanny is so endearing and affectionate that the adolescents still kiss her good-bye every time she leaves their home. Clearly, this mother is especially privileged to have encountered a sincere and loving substitute caregiver for her children. Like the minority of children who receive excellent and high quality day care, these young twins are cared for devotedly by a special caregiver in their home.

MATERNAL DEPRIVATION SYNDROME

As a rule, the healthy development of young children is taken for granted. The development of young children, however, is complex and specific. Ashley Montagu (1996b, 97) describes the following significant developmental periods during childhood:

1. The first period begins at birth and is established by five to six months of age. During this period the infant is establishing a cooperative relationship with a clearly defined person—the mother.

2. The second period continues through the end of the third year and is characterized by the child's need for the mother to be constantly available.

3. The third period occurs during the fourth and fifth years and is marked by the child's ability to maintain a relationship with the mother despite her absence for a few days or perhaps a few weeks

Clearly, the presence and availability of the mother is very critical to these developmental periods.

A mother's absence in her young child's life results in a disruption of these developmental periods. This interference may affect a young child's maturation process adversely. Ashley Montagu (1996b, 98) offers keen insight into the type of behavior that may ensue when the critical developmental periods are disrupted:

> Unless the child has been firmly grounded in the discipline of love and interdependency, he is damaged in his ability to develop clear and definite judgments concerning people and things, and his ability to form such judgments as an adult is seriously handicapped. As adults the judgments of such persons tend to be blurred and vague. Their decisions about the world, people and things tend to be characterized by doubt, suspicion, uncertainty, misgiving and unsureness. They vacillate, in short, they tend to see the world through a mist of unshed tears. They are characterized by an inability to enter into the feelings of others because, when they were young, no one cared enough to enter into theirs.

In other words, the child who experiences the disruption of these critical developmental periods has difficulty establishing a firm foundation of wisdom in his life. Evidently, a child develops the ability to judge and make decisions from early infancy in the presence of a consistent and loving caregiver.

There is little doubt that an individual's inability to make clear judgments as an older child and adult is a significant liability. This lack of wisdom puts these children and adults in a vulnerable position. Undoubtedly, all human beings make errors, but healthy and sensible individuals eventually learn from their mistakes and develop better judgment. Among those who lack good judgment, some are lucky enough to avoid experiencing deep trouble while others may not be able to learn from their errors.

For example, I am well acquainted with an adult who has been a lifelong drug addict. He is an intelligent and talented man, and he once articulated to me what he perceived to be his problem. He told me that if his mother had breastfed him, he would never have turned out as he did. I did not appreciate the significance of his remark until many years later. His comment was profoundly insightful, and it reflected his awareness of his problem. Unfortunately, he could not nurture greater wisdom and use common sense to avoid using illicit drugs. My friend was denied sensory pleasure as an infant and young child; he has not recovered from the deprivation even though he is now in his fifties.

As more individuals experience maternal deprivation and fail to develop a foundation of wisdom in their lives, they will undoubtedly need to cultivate greater wisdom on their own later in life. This may be difficult to accomplish when one's peers are similarly as unwise and deficient in common sense. Ultimately, it is maternal deprivation, and not lack of parental influence, that explains why some children are more susceptible to the pressure and negative influence of their peers. These are also the same children who often disregard their parents' wisdom and advice.

Ultimately, it is not that parental care is meaningless in child development, as Harris absurdly suggests. Rather, it is impossible for children to value parental influence when such influence was absent in early childhood. In comparison, when children receive an abundance of loving maternal care early in life, they will be able to experience the opposite of maternal deprivation syndrome: they will almost assuredly develop the ability to think soundly.

My son, for instance, has shown me repeatedly that he can think soundly on his own. I can still recall an astounding experience in which he gave me a dirty look when he was only nine months old. I had initiated an argument with my husband and instead of resolving my differences with him, I persisted in bickering. My son's assessment of the situation was very clear: I was the culprit who was unnecessarily protracting the argument. As an infant, my son had already developed a keen sense of judgment.

When babies and young children are nurtured well, they will develop the strength of character and self-identity that will permit them to judge the influence of their peers and their parents fairly and meaningfully. In other words, it is less likely that peers will exert a harmful influence upon a child who has been nurtured in the bosom of a loving and caring family with breastfeeding. Breastfeeding and the provision of loving maternal care cannot be ignored any longer if parents care to matter in their children's lives.

WOMEN CHOOSE NOT TO STAY HOME

Despite what would seem to be a natural inclination for women to choose to stay home to mother their young infants, many women do not. A record high of 59 percent of mothers with infants were in the labor force in 1998 (O'Connell 2001). This means that millions of young babies who are too young to walk do not receive the benefits of hands-on maternal care. One may surmise from this statistic that the majority of parents think that maternal care is unnecessary, impractical, or perhaps unimportant.

I know parents who have made this assumption for differing reasons. I once surprised a pregnant friend by asking her if she would leave her job to care for her newborn. Such a possibility apparently had not crossed her mind since she was her family's primary breadwinner. My friend had worked for the same company for many years, and she had no intention of giving up either her senior position or her work benefits. After a short maternity leave, my friend resumed her regular work schedule and placed her daughter in an in-home day care center in her neighborhood.

I also knew a couple who had researched day care options for their newborn. They were delighted to enroll their young infant at the age of six weeks into a school. This couple insisted that their daughter was attending school, and not day care, at a cost of $10,000 per year. Their conviction that this was the best option seemed to overlook the possibility that the baby's mother could afford to stay home with the child since the father was developing a successful dental practice.

In both cases, each family assumed that their young infants would do as well as or perhaps even better in day care than they would have had they received maternal care in the home. One should wonder from where this kind of assumption arises. Dr. Elliott Barker in Canada, a physician who has worked extensively with the criminally insane, has called day care "the biggest unproved experiment of the twentieth century." The assumption that day care is equivalent to maternal care at home is terribly misleading since numerous studies have shown that the greater majority of institutional and in-home day care centers fail to provide young infants the correct stimulation for their healthy growth and development.

My friend and the couple were fortunate to have found excellent day care facilities for their newborns. My friend is scrupulously attentive to the details of her daughter's care, and the couple was willing to pay for high quality day care. Undoubtedly, they screened their children's day care centers for quality, care, safety, and educational enrichment. This probably meant that the day care providers were organized and capable of managing the care of many babies and children simultaneously. It is hard to trust, nevertheless, that a day care worker who is responsible for the care of four to eight young babies and young children concurrently could provide attention remotely similar to the kind of care that a mother could offer one baby or even a few children of different ages in the home.

10

ANY CARE BUT MATERNAL CARE

DISTORTED VIEWS OF INFANT DEVELOPMENT

Even though maternal care has been crucial to the well-being of children and family throughout human history, hands-on maternal care is no longer thought to be practical. This biased view of maternal care is disseminated specifically by day care researchers and journalists who promote day care as being the single reasonable answer to what they perceive to be the problem of child care. Although the goal of day care research should be to determine the positive and negative effects of day care upon the well-being of young children and the family unit, published studies related to day care research are rarely objective.

For instance, psychologist Sandra Scarr is a leading day care researcher who published numerous studies and articles that were always in support of day care throughout the 1980s and the 1990s. During many of the years she published her pro-day care studies and articles in academic journals and mainstream publications, Scarr had close ties to KinderCare Inc., a nationwide chain of for-profit day care franchises in the U.S. She served on KinderCare's board from 1990; was elected Chairman of the Board in 1994; and was made Chief Executive Officer in 1995, at which time she left the faculty of the University of Virginia but continued to publish pro-day care articles in academic journals (Robertson 2003, 108).

In the November 7, 1987, issue of the *Washington Post*, Sandra Evans quotes Scarr as saying that the brains of infants "are Jell-O and their memories akin to decorticate rodents." Scarr posits that "only the most pervasive and disastrous experiences during early infancy would have any long-term negative effect on development." Sandra Scarr's remarks have been and are still publicized widely even though her line of reasoning is flawed: there is no objective evidence at all that suggests that the memories of babies can be compared to that of brain-damaged rodents.

Even so, views of infant care similar to that promoted by Scarr have abounded for many decades. For instance, one of the most basic and cruel premises of infants' experience of pain has been to assume that babies do not feel pain. Thus, countless parents have been informed that a baby can tolerate the pain of undergoing procedures like circumcision, blood drawing, and immunizations without the need for anesthesia.

Innumerable newborn boys have experienced and continue to undergo circumcision without receiving any pain relief. The babies scream and cry vigorously as their foreskins are removed surgically, their skin bleeds, and their genitalia look raw and unnaturally exposed. This sight may horrify parents and engender sympathy, but they continue to trust that their babies do not experience pain. The same adults, however, will wince with pain over a simple paper cut.

Parents are also informed that their newborns and young infants will suffer just a small bit as they are subjected to painful procedures like blood drawing and immunizations without the administration of anesthesia. About a decade ago, the issue of pain relief for childhood immunizations was finally addressed when a topical anesthetic was made available to dull the pain of receiving an injection. Meanwhile, more studies are finding that infants and children most certainly do experience pain, and they are not as resilient and immune to suffering as physicians and psychologists claimed they were. Contrary to the callous and unscientific assumptions of psychologists like Scarr, it is evident that even minor experiences of pain and suffering can interfere with healthy human development.

Guidelines to limit pain in newborns were published in the February 2001 issue of *Archives of Pediatric and Adolescent Medicine* (Anand et al. 2001). The authors of the study observed the following: "Compared with older children and adults, neonates are more sensitive to pain and vulnerable to its long-term effects. Despite the clinical importance of neonatal pain, current medical practices continue to expose infants to repetitive, acute, or prolonged pain." The authors, according to an article in Reuters Health on February 21, 2005, recommend greater awareness of pain in the newborn period because adequate pain treatment can "not only improve the clinical care provided to all neonates, but may also have a positive impact on their subsequent health and behaviors during childhood and adolescence."

Another study in *Lancet* stated that pain experienced in the newborn period could have a long-lasting impact upon later infant behavior. The study's authors (Taddio et al. 1997) came to the following conclusion:

> The results of this study are consistent with studies of pain response in animals and behavioural studies in humans showing that injury and tissue damage sustained in infancy can cause sustained changes in central neural function, which persist after the wound has healed and influence behavioural responses to painful events months later. Pretreatment and postoperative management of neonatal circumcision pain is recommended based on these results. Investigation of the neurological basis of these effects is warranted.

The authors' findings contradict Sandra Scarr's unscientific view of infant development. If anything, studies demonstrate that infants experience greater pain and suffering than do older children and adults.

Scarr's assumption that infants do not experience profound and long-term negative effects from less than disastrous experiences is wrong. She has published enough misinformation, however, to lead millions of parents to trust that any care is sufficient for their babies. Moreover, as an expert in the field of day care research, Scarr has undoubtedly influenced her fellow researchers.

Sandra Evans quotes Scarr in the *Washington Post* as saying the following at a conference of day care researchers: "Infancy is so protected by biological design…it is hard to throw them [infants] off for very long." Sandra Scarr should qualify her understanding of what it means to "throw" off an infant from the course of healthy human development. One may surmise that Scarr's perception of the course of an infant's healthy human development is set to an unbelievably low standard. What else can one expect, however, from a psychologist who compares infants' brains to Jell-O?

BIAS TOWARD DAY CARE

Journalist Tom Zoellner wrote a thoroughly researched article about the lack of objectivity many researchers and academicians demonstrate toward the analysis of day care studies. Sandra Scarr is one of numerous day care researchers and journalists who are outspoken advocates of day care; many of them are women who have placed their own children in day care. Prominent day care researchers and journalists who publicize the research are candid about their pro-day care bias.

Leading day care researcher Alison Clarke-Stewart, for instance, relays the following to Zoellner (2001): "Maternal employment is a reality. The issue today, therefore, is not whether infants should be in day care but how to make their experiences there and at home supportive of their development and of their parents' peace of mind." Day care advocates do not consider the possibility of providing infants with maternal care. All that matters is that parents should find sufficiently decent day care for their babies since this will enable mothers who work outside the home to be assured "peace of mind."

Researchers like Scarr and Clarke-Stewart are biased, and they do not offer objective views of day care. The same can be said of the journalists who promote the widespread dissemination of misinformation about the real consequences of day care. The politically correct and pro-day care stance of the media is focused single-mindedly on supporting a woman's right to work outside the home. Consequently, there is little or no regard for either the young children who need maternal care or the women who wish to care for their own children.

The media tend to glorify any study that purports to show that non-maternal care is suitable for all children. In 1999, for instance, many newspapers and journals cited uncritically a study by Elizabeth Harvey that claimed that children in day care were unharmed by receiving non-maternal care. Without researching the background or the validity of the study, the media used Harvey's conclusion to report to the general public that working women had no need to worry about the well-being of children who had been placed in any care but maternal care.

According to Zoellner, the basis of the study is a huge ongoing government survey, the National Longitudinal Survey of Youth (NLSY), in which people are interviewed every few years. The data base was not directed specifically toward evaluating day care, and the survey respondents did not represent a broad sampling of middle-class Americans. Instead, the subjects surveyed had half the average American income, half were minority, half were single women, the median IQ of 80 was lower than the average American IQ of 100, the mothers were younger than the average childbearing American mother, and the mothers' assessments of their children's emotional state were not verified objectively.

David Murray, a statistician who assists journalists in deciphering complicated mathematical data, informs Zoellner that Harvey "crunched her numbers in such a way that it would make any ill effects of mothers' employment very hard to detect" (Zoellner 2005). When contacted by Zoellner, Harvey acknowledges that the study had limitations, which she had noted in the study, and that the data obtained from the group surveyed "may not be generalized to older, higher socioeconomic parents." She did not, however, volunteer the limitations of her study to reporters. At the time of Zoellner's interview, Harvey was pregnant and planning to place her infant in day care.

In the meantime, Zoellner learns that Jay Belsky, a psychologist and well-known day care researcher, had difficulty getting his study published in the same journal that published Harvey's faulty study. Belsky had alienated himself from the world of day care studies because he had concluded that too many hours in day care may lead infants to develop impaired relations with their parents and demonstrate behavioral problems later in childhood. Belsky's findings apparently did not accord with the views of influential day care researchers and journalists who promote day care with unbridled optimism.

Journalist Sue Shellenbarger, for instance, is a mother of five children who wrote a column called "Work and Family" in the *Wall Street Journal* in June 1999. She summarized her understanding of a massive study called the National Institute of Child Health and Human Development (NICHHD) project. According to Zoellner, even the project's researchers could not agree on the significance of all the data they had accumulated. This did not deter Shellenbarger, however, from concluding the following: "Kids in high-quality child care settings, as gauged by care-giver sensitivity, responsiveness and conversation, did better than all other children, even those in their mother's care, on cognitive and language tests" (Zoellner 2001).

Shellenbarger's interpretation of the data and her assertion that high quality child care was superior to maternal care is absurd. As a journalist, she must have known that the chances of finding such high quality day care are minimal. Also, according to Zoellner, Shellenbarger's "own experiences with day care have run the gamut from high-quality to abysmal—a sort of NICHHD study in microcosm."

One is left to conclude that since Shellenbarger's five children tolerated inconsistent day care experiences, it will be similarly acceptable for many other women's children to experience the same range of high-quality to appallingly bad care. Shellenbarger's interpretation of the NICHHD study was widely publicized and is still cited by day care advocates to support their unfounded argument that day care provides children with greater benefits than maternal care. Surely, there are exceptional cases in which babies would do better in day care, but the broad assumption that all mothers can and should abdicate their responsibility in child-rearing is ridiculous.

Astoundingly enough, pro-day care propaganda appears to exist simply because women want to hear positive affirmation of their decision to place their young babies in day care. For instance, Zoellner (2001) quotes Clarke-Stewart as saying, "I wanted to find out that child care was good. I'm a working mother, but that's not the only reason. It made common sense to me."

Other women are less biased. Thus, Marilyn Elias, a journalist who covers day care for *USA Today*, offers this view of day care: "It's a topic that engenders emotion in both researchers and reporters. It's not played straight. There are reporters who play it fairly and those who don't. Take it all with a grain of salt. It always pays to do your own independent research. Follow your gut as a parent. It's being filtered through somebody's eyes" (Zoellner 2001).

It is evident that objective day care researchers and journalists may address a baby's existence with sentiments that border on apathy. Their curious indifference to the well-being of young children contrasts sharply with their relentless and passionate support of day care. Regrettably, the influence this minority of women wields is enormous. Harvey's report, for instance, was disseminated widely. Zoellner notes that Harvey was interviewed by over fifty news sources, including top television stations and newspapers, all of whom accepted her conclusions without reservations.

It is deplorable that anyone, particularly those who play a role in educating the general public, would proffer misleading and overly optimistic pronouncements about the resilience and adaptability of young babies and children. It is sad and unconscionable that the perennially positive or neutral presentation of day care to the general public deludes millions of parents into trusting that they do not need to provide maternal care for their young babies. Currently, far too many young babies and children do not receive consistent maternal care. Granted, there are parents who are unable to offer their children maternal care, but there are many more parents who could but do not because they trust that maternal care in the modern era is obsolete.

The reality is that parents who trust that day care is fine for their children are playing "Russian roulette with a generation," as Jay Belsky informs Sandra Evans of the *Washington Post*. Simply stated, the adamantly pro-day care advocates offer advice to parents that does not correlate with the reality of the day care situation in the U.S. The current day care system for the majority of young babies and children does not provide the intimate care that maternal care can provide.

Sadly, day care advocates do not seem to appreciate on even the most basic level the importance of maternal care in young children's development. Instead, they assert repeatedly the right of women to work outside the home and the government's obligation to provide suitable and affordable day care facilities for the numerous young babies and children who do not receive maternal care. Ultimately, day care advocates will face the same situation as the many other parents who trust that the withholding of maternal care in early childhood will not impair their children's development or their relationship with them.

Countless thousands of parents already need guidance to relate to their uncommunicative and sullen children. This reality is reflected in the growth of services offered by various types of corrective behavioral camps all over the country. These boot camps are harsh and punitive environments that force youngsters, some barely in their teens, to learn the meaning of discipline and respect, perhaps at the cost of their lives. Such dehumanizing approaches to child-rearing have arisen as a result of the inability of parents and children to relate to and communicate with one another.

The fact that millions of children are no longer receiving intimate maternal care means that such businesses will continue to thrive, even though they have not been shown to ameliorate the suffering of children and parents who fail to communicate with one another meaningfully. In the meantime, pro-day care advocates can claim that they are not responsible for parents' decision to withhold maternal care. After all, parents are intelligent and capable of making sound decisions on their own. In other words, pro-day care advocates will be unavailable and unable to offer meaningful words of wisdom to the millions of parents who trust the bias against maternal care.

Meanwhile, day care advocates will not take responsibility for the biased nature of their research and reporting because it only made sense to them, as Clarke-Stewart would say. Day care research, however, as it is performed and reported in the modern era does not make sense at all. It is biased, and it rarely considers the well-being of either children or their parents. The irony is that the promotion of day care is supposed to help women to fulfill their various roles in life, but there is one unique womanly role that is excluded: the role of hands-on mother. The consequences of ignoring the maternal role in child-rearing are becoming more evident daily, and the news is not good.

THE RISK OF DISREGARDING MATERNAL CARE

Susan Chira of the *New York Times* reports on February 7, 1995, that a study entitled "Cost, Quality and Child Outcomes in Child Care Centers" is the "latest of several condemning the quality of American child care, whether in centers or in family day care, where one adult cares for a small group of children in a home." The study was conducted by child psychologists and economists at four universities who examined 400 care centers in California, Colorado, Connecticut, and North Carolina in the spring of 1993. The researchers found that "overall, 12 percent of the centers were unsafe or unsanitary, and only 1 in 7 offered the kind of warm relationships that teach children how to trust adults and the intellectual stimulation that helps children become ready for school." Jay Belsky, then a professor of human development at Pennsylvania State University, is quoted as saying that "the problem is that good care is so scarce."

Robert Lee Hotz of the *Los Angeles Times* reports on October 28, 1997, in "Neglect Harms Infants' Brains, Researchers Say" that research on Romanian orphans raised in state-run wards shows that "parental care makes such a lasting impression on an infant that maternal separation or neglect can profoundly affect the brain's biochemistry, with lifelong consequences for growth and mental ability." Hotz also writes that "new animal research reveals that without the attention of a loving caregiver early in life, some of an infant's brain cells may simply commit suicide." Analyzing the effects of maternal deprivation in laboratory animals at the DuPont Merck Research Labs, psychologist Mark Smith said his research team was shocked to learn that "maternal separation caused these cells in the [infant] brain to die." Smith surmises that the "effects of maternal deprivation may be much more profound" than researchers had suspected.

An article by Melissa Faye Greene in the June 17, 2000, issue of the *New Yorker* magazine highlights different outcomes for various children who are adopted from abroad after having experienced institutionalized care in their homeland. For example, one American couple adopts a boy from a Russian orphanage when he is twenty-one months old. An initial evaluation correlates his development to be comparable to that of a twelve-month-old baby. His adoptive parents exert themselves tirelessly and lovingly on his behalf and enroll him in a special-needs school. It takes approximately two years for the child to become securely attached to his adoptive parents. By the time he is four years old, he is assessed to be a gifted child, and he embraces his recently adopted nine-month-old baby sister who is also from Russia.

In contrast to the success of this couple with their adopted children is the case of the Hannons, a couple who adopts a Romanian orphan when she is three years old. At age eleven, cognitive tests assess her development to be comparable to that of a three-year-old. Greene notes that eleven-year-old Juliana has stunted growth, grimaces and rocks, has never spoken a word, and is not completely toilet trained. Her adoptive parents were assured that the child would be cured with love and time, but the child has shown practically no signs of recovering from her early childhood deprivation.

Juliana has received several diagnoses over the years, including "post-traumatic stress disorder, pervasive development disorder, institutional autism, and brain injury" (Greene 2000). Her adoptive mother sums up their daughter's condition by remarking insightfully that her daughter "fits a lot of categories. But the bottom line is that she's a kid who spent three years in an institution." Her adoptive mother has started a support group, the Parent Network for the Post-Institutionalized Child, with another parent of a troubled Romanian child.

Ultimately, deprivation in early childhood can have long-lasting and deleterious effects upon children's growth and development. Whether or not these effects can be reversed is questionable. There is certainly a matter of chance and fortune involved in many of these cases. The Russian boy and girl were resilient enough to withstand the deprivation of early childhood. In contrast, Juliana could not adapt to the love and embrace offered by dedicated and caring adoptive parents who had improved immeasurably the quality of her life. It is discouraging to realize that the Hannons were unable to reverse the effects of the deprivation Juliana experienced during early childhood.

The plight of the Romanian orphans helped to publicize the gravity of maternal deprivation syndrome and its consequences in the late 1990s. Awareness of maternal deprivation syndrome, however, has subsided significantly in recent years. The majority of American parents are undoubtedly confident that their children will never suffer as the Romanian orphans have. After all, the majority of American parents love their children and would never purposefully subject their young babies to conditions remotely similar to those faced by orphans in Romanian institutions.

In the present era, however, millions of young babies and children no longer receive maternal care. It is assumed de facto that babies and children will do fine in the absence of maternal care. What else are parents to think when day care researchers and journalists repeatedly offer a positive outlook on day care?

Pro-day care advocates are doing an insidiously effective job of convincing far too many parents that maternal care is passé and insignificant. Even as they make pronouncements about young children's resilience and their ability to withstand great adversity, it is simply too facile to assume that children will not suffer as a result of receiving insufficient maternal care. At the same time, one should wonder how women, including Scarr and Clarke-Stewart, could so easily forget the uniqueness of a woman's role in her child's life.

HOW WOMEN FORGOT THE ART OF MOTHERING

Much of the bias against stay-at-home mothering can be attributed to the persistent image of a mythical creation of the entertainment industry: the ebullient and domesticated 1950s housewife. For some perverse reason, the modern perception of motherhood is indelibly attached to the failings and disappointments associated with the 1950s housewife. Conservatives and liberals alike persist narrow-mindedly in restricting their vision of human mothering to the 1950s era.

The 1950s is often remembered by conservatives as being a golden era for child-rearing and family life, partly for good reasons. Through the GI Bill, the U.S. government offered significant financial support that enabled millions of World War II veterans to pursue education, including college, and purchase their own homes. Corporations in that era were also more loyal to both blue-collar and white-collar employees. Such benefits and job security permitted untold numbers of men to support their stay-at-home wives and children.

From another perspective, however, it is well known that the 1950s was also a time when substance abuse was common among adults. Alcoholism was the norm among both men and women: alcohol was served and drunk during a long lunch hour, the cocktail hour, before and after dinner, and as a nightcap. Cigarette smoking was also prevalent, even among pregnant women. Many women were also prescribed anti-anxiety medications. Irrespective of the post-war prosperity that should have benefited women and family life, there is no doubt that neither women nor their families were truly healthy. Thus, to glorify the 1950s as being a perfect era for child-rearing is disingenuous and simply wrong.

By the middle of the twentieth century, women were unable to rear their children as independently and confidently as their predecessors. Many women were uprooted from their extended families and, with their husbands away at work, young mothers were left to care for their babies alone. These women may have been alone, but they were not independent and self-sufficient since motherly intuition and wisdom had already been displaced by an unnatural dependency upon the guidance of child-rearing experts decades earlier.

Although parenting books had been around in some form or other for centuries, the influence of parenting books intensified at the turn of the twentieth century. In 1894 pediatrician Luther Emmett Holt wrote a child-rearing guide called *The Care and Feeding of Children: A Catechism for the Use of Mothers and Children's Nurses*. It was a guide that would be read by millions of mothers and mothers-to-be for over fifty years, making Holt the "Dr. Spock" of his day (Montagu 1986, 148).

Holt's influence has been long-lasting and still taints current American child-rearing practices. He recommended regimented parenting practices, including not picking up babies when they cried, enforcing rigid feeding schedules, using stationary cribs instead of rocking cradles, and not actively promoting breastfeeding (Montagu 1986, 99). Child-rearing, according to Holt, was to be centered upon the premise that young infants were innately willful creatures who needed to be raised in a strict and unloving manner.

The reverberations of such an unhealthy philosophy of child-rearing continue to influence parents to this day. Holt's legacy lives on in numerous books by other child-rearing experts, many of whom do not seem to understand how healthy and loving human beings develop. Currently, there are many books that espouse the unenlightened and damaging philosophy of child-rearing experts who misunderstand young children.

Whereas women throughout history were the primary physicians, healers, and nurturers of their families, many women are now unsure about nearly everything related to the well-being of young children. It is not the fault of women today that they are no longer the confident and able mothers they once were. A mother's role as nurturer of her children has been in a state of profound confusion for decades.

PUTTING BABIES FIRST

A young baby needs a responsive caregiver to be available at all times, and the ideal person to provide such care is the baby's mother. This may not be possible for every family in today's society, but it is something that can and should be considered seriously. If parents would like to nurture their children's unique potentialities, then they should contemplate the profound significance of breastfeeding and stay-at-home mothering.

Over the past several years, particularly among highly educated and married women, women have begun to choose to stay home to care for young children. This trend is confirmed by a small drop in the percentage of women with infants in the workforce, which decreased from a high of 59 percent in 1998 to 55 percent in 2000 (O'Connell 2001). Women who choose to stay home are not being forced to stay home: it is the opposite, in fact. In a 1998 survey done by a women's group called Mothers and More, 89% of respondents cited the statement "I wanted to raise my children myself" as the primary reason for choosing to stay home with their children (American Demographics 2002).

The premise that women would want to stay home to breastfeed and mother their babies, unfortunately, irks a vocal minority of women who have for many decades either dismissed or spoken out against the importance of breastfeeding and stay-at-home mothering. They view mother-infant bonding as being both abnormal and a scientific myth. Consequently, a woman who stays home may need to defend her decision to stay home with her children.

Over the years I have stayed home, I have encountered several stay-at-home mothers who seem to shrink when they comment on their homemaking. I once overheard a woman exclaim that she has no talents at all and that she just stays home. In the meantime, she runs a business from her home, and she is a busy and cheerful volunteer at her daughter's school. Granted, few women burst forth with unbridled enthusiasm when commenting on their homemaking, but there is no need for women to disparage themselves. Even so, women may find that they need to defend their choice to stay home with their young children.

It is evident that many women are confused about the role they should play in their young children's lives. This is to be expected since a woman's role in family life is rarely mentioned or considered in modern education. Education today is centered upon fostering individualism and the search for self-identity. Thus, young women and men are advised to discover their specific talents, reach for their personal dreams, and enter any profession or occupation they desire. This type of formal schooling trains the next generation of workers and consumers, but it does little to encourage the development of humane and caring parents.

On the whole, modern education fails to help students develop any concept of the importance of family life and the unique function of parents in child-rearing. The lack of exposure to and the dearth of discussion about family life in modern education impair the ability of many young adults to think independently and critically of current child-rearing practices. Uninformed and perhaps uninterested, individuals often trust that the norms of child-rearing, including the abandonment of a baby's care to anyone other than his mother, are unobjectionable.

It is difficult to blame parents for following the modern trend of baby care since most child-rearing experts appear to deny the significance of maternal care. Their advice generally emphasizes the resilience of a young baby; his ability to be alone and comfort himself; the need for a mother to let go of her attachment to her baby (as if there is something pathologically wrong with loving one's baby); the need for a mother to return to a life of normalcy (as if the baby does not exist); and the need for a baby to get to know people (almost anyone, in fact) other than his mother, the one person a baby needs most. This advice convinces parents that their young babies and children can adapt to whatever experiences life brings them. It is almost as if mothers and fathers can ignore the essential and irreplaceable roles they play in their children's lives.

One should question, however, what has happened to the parental role of protecting one's baby and cherishing the life of the unique individual who was born to a specific set of parents. In light of the extreme immaturity of the human infant, mothers should be able to provide hands-on maternal care for at least the first five to six years of a child's life. On the contrary, most parents have learned incorrectly that breastfeeding and maternal care are not integral aspects of healthy child-rearing practices.

As a result, in the year 2005, a minority of women are stay-at-home mothers, and those who also breastfeed their babies for more than six months comprise an even smaller minority. Women today are busy and, understandably, some can barely manage to fit their children into their busy schedules. Parents may even take pride in doing so much that parenting may become another life activity that needs to be squeezed into one's busy schedule. For some women, then, mothering may become another item of accomplishment to be checked off at the end of the day.

THE MYTH OF PARENTAL FREEDOM

It is unfortunate that the myth of parental freedom encourages parents to disengage themselves from even young babies. Mainstream publications, particularly women's magazines, promote frequently the need for parents to recapture the sparkle of romance that existed before a baby's birth. Ironically, they use celebrities to glorify dating and romancing over parenting even though celebrities are notorious for divorcing and being less than ideal parenting role models.

In the name of promoting healthier marriages but not necessarily better parenting skills, parents are encouraged to return to dating and leave their children behind. The food service industry, the entertainment industry, and baby-sitters may delight that dating parents spend more money, but one must wonder about the young babies and children who are left behind. Is it worthwhile for a couple to see a movie together and dine out, for instance, while their small infant stays home with a babysitter?

An article in the April 25, 2005, issue of *Newsweek* offers parents the following advice: "Research shows that the better your marriage is, the better off your child will be—academically and socially" (Robb 2005, 48). This guidance makes sense since stable family situations, which include healthy marriages, invariably support more optimal child development. This statement, however, is made in the context of an article that suggests that parents who wish to live "happily ever after" should "get a babysitter." The nefarious assumption is that children may fare worse developmentally if parents do not spend time alone and away from their children. It is curious that parents are urged to spend time away from their young children exactly at a time when they are needed the most.

There is a timeline for everything, and parents can perhaps enjoy the freedom of doing things other than child-rearing when their young children no longer need their consistent presence. Additionally, one should consider what freedom is. Ashley Montagu (1996a, 76) offers the following pertinent description: "…freedom does not consist in the liberty to do what we like, but in the right to be able to do what we ought." Sadly, it has become politically incorrect to suggest that parents should reconsider the concept of freedom and realize that responsibility is integral to true freedom.

THE NOT SO BENIGN NEGLECT OF BABIES

In recent years, it has become evident that parents may forget that they are caring for highly dependent babies and children. Within the past two years in Southern California, two infants died of heatstroke after they were left unattended for hours in hot and unventilated cars. The cases were unrelated, but the scenarios were nearly identical.

The fathers of the two babies were supposed to drop their babies off at day care on their way to work. Instead, the fathers parked their cars, went to work, and forgot about their babies. These tragic cases point out how easily one can forget one's responsibilities as a parent when intimate maternal care is not the norm. These fathers simply forgot that they were responsible for their babies' care. In contrast, it is inconceivable that a breastfeeding mother would ever forget to attend to her infant since she is biologically bound to her.

Although the birth of babies should bring about great changes in parental lifestyles, some parents are unable or unwilling to make significant lifestyle alterations. The care of a baby may become merely another daily errand that consists of dropping the baby off at a day care center or making sure the nanny arrives on time. While the baby's well-being is entrusted to day care workers or nannies, parents are free to fulfill responsibilities other than parenting. In these situations, a baby's presence in her parents' lives may be so unusual that a parent could actually forget the baby's existence. One has to wonder, however, what kinds of experiences young infants endure when parents can possibly forget their babies' existence.

Babies should receive the consistent intimacy, warmth, and comfort of loving and available maternal care. This does not mean that a baby is constantly bombarded with loving smiles and coos from an overly attentive mother. Rather, a baby becomes an integral part of her mother's life so that the baby experiences the reality of her mother's existence. A baby is held in her mother's arms while she does various things inside and outside the home. She is nearby while her mother cooks and does the myriad things that need to be accomplished each day. Additionally, a baby can also experience the pleasure of being breastfed and cradled.

Simply put, a baby can enjoy being with her mother. This kind of experience, however, is not the norm for most babies. In contrast, too many babies awaken early in the morning for the simple objective of being dropped off at day care or placed in the care of someone other than mother. Ultimately, one has to question if babies today receive sufficient intimacy and loving affection. It is becoming apparent that current child-rearing practices are leading many babies to experience frustration, hunger, anger, and helplessness as normal conditions of life.

Susan Cheever writes in the *New Yorker* magazine about the conditions under which nannies worked for middle-class and upper middle-class families in Manhattan during the mid-1990s. She interviews nannies whom she describes as being sensible, caring, capable, and concerned. Cheever (1995, 87) quotes one nanny, Sally, as saying, "Sometimes it blows me away when I'll come in to work and there will be no milk and no cereal and no money for groceries. Two people without kids, who eat out don't have to have groceries, but with kids you need to have something for them to eat."

Cheever offers a comparable description of the eating habits of the employers of Dominique, another nanny: "The people she works for eat out, and the children live on sweet cereal, bread, boxed fruit juice, and peanut butter and jelly that are premixed in the jar" (85). Also, even though the younger child is eight months old, he is still drinking only infant formula because the "employer seems reluctant to give up the ease and convenience of four-ounce nursettes—prefilled bottles" (85). The article provides fairly concrete evidence that the young children of even financially well-off and highly educated parents experience frustration often and unnecessarily.

The neglect these young children experience indicates how unaware many parents are about their young children's development as human beings. It is hypocritical to deny young babies the fulfillment of basic needs while parents seek satisfaction in their own lives. Naturally, there will be times when a young baby has to wait for fulfillment since even the most obliging and loving breastfeeding mother will not always be available. Nevertheless, to make babies experience disappointment and dissatisfaction regularly is both cruel and irresponsible.

THE MOTHER-INFANT DIVIDE

It would be more reasonable to establish a secure foundation of love and satisfaction in a young baby's life so that he will be able to weather the vicissitudes of uncertainty that will occur later in life. Contrary to current ideology, early childhood should revolve around satisfaction, and breastfeeding can provide such fulfillment while simultaneously offering the baby a positive understanding of healthy human interaction and intimacy.

The reality, however, is that many babies are fed infant formula, and they do not receive the intimacy of breastfeeding. The ingestion of infant formula should be an enjoyable experience, but many parents and caregivers do not even bother to pick up their babies to feed them infant formula. They either prop up the bottles or make babies hold their own bottles. Consequently, babies may experience drinking infant formula not only as a tedious and joyless activity but also as one that does not offer much intimacy or meaningful interaction with a loving caregiver.

At the same time, many parents are convinced that a baby needs to suck, so they plug their baby's mouth with a pacifier. Even though a baby would prefer to suckle at the breast, parents may encourage their baby to suck on a pacifier. Despite its inconvenience, since a pacifier usually falls out of a baby's mouth repeatedly, parents become accustomed to placing the pacifier in their baby's mouth. Thus, the baby is trained to attach herself to a pacifier instead of enabling her to interact meaningfully with her mother.

Much of this trend in infant care, wherein the distance between a mother and her baby is encouraged, has to do with the glorification and prioritization of a woman's need to achieve greater personal fulfillment. A woman may be a mother, but it has become unacceptable to associate womanly happiness with mothering alone. Increasingly, women feel compelled to distinguish themselves as having occupations and preoccupations other than mothering. Although women have every right to pursue personal fulfillment, one should wonder how much true satisfaction a woman gains by detaching herself from her infant.

About a decade ago one of my friends was pregnant with her first child when she decided to pursue further study in medicine. Her mother came to care for the baby, and my friend started her fellowship. After a few months, the baby's grandmother needed to leave, so my friend hired help through a nanny placement service. From the outset, the nanny was apathetic and callously unattached to my friend's infant son.

By all appearances, my friend's baby managed to survive this nanny's unpleasant care and demeanor for a year. As a pre-schooler, however, he experienced the sudden and inexplicable loss of all his bodily hair. Over the course of two years, the child was taken to various specialists who examined him, prescribed different treatments, and could not identify the cause of the hair loss. Luckily for the boy and his parents, his hair eventually grew back. Although the boy was able to recover, there is little doubt that he and his parents suffered greatly from this ordeal.

Irrespective of the gentle, loving, and kind demeanor of my friend and her husband, their little boy's caregiver subjected him to insensitive indifference or perhaps cruel care. The little boy's hair loss most likely reflected the severe stress his nervous system experienced in the hands of an unloving and apathetic caregiver. Ashley Montagu (1986, 5) describes the inextricable connection between the skin and the nervous system: "The nervous system is, then, a buried part of the skin, or alternatively the skin may be regarded as an exposed portion of the nervous system."

The reality is that it is impossible to predict the consequences of denying young children devoted maternal care. Parents may argue that they need to find fulfillment in their lives first and that they will help to satisfy their children's needs eventually but not necessarily during early childhood. For instance, a neighbor of mine once explained why she was certain that her young babies did not need her care. She said, "They don't need me now. They'll need me later when they're in school."

My neighbor trusted that a nanny could do everything as well as she could to meet her babies' needs for nourishment, sleep, warmth, cleanliness, and other bodily care. She intimated that she could communicate better with her children once they were older. Thus, a nanny cared for my neighbor's two young children while she pursued work outside the home and waited for the time when her children would truly need her.

11

MOTHERS

WOMEN AND MODERN EDUCATION

Some women have argued persuasively that they cannot be good mothers if they are neither happy nor fulfilled. They contend that the primary way in which they feel content and satisfied is by working outside the home. The concurrent and underlying argument is that women cannot be happy if they stay home and care for their children.

It is not surprising that the movement to expel women from the home and into the workforce is as strong as it is. Over the last several decades, the majority of women have been educated in institutions that were originally designed to educate men. In an essay written originally in 1958, Ashley Montagu (1967, 206) offers this astute analysis of modern education:

> It is through the agency of education, particularly college education, that women have been especially trained in a confused perception of their roles. The chief error has been to educate women as if they were men. In most of our schools and colleges there is scarcely any recognition given to the fact that such a difference as male and female exists. In most of our women's colleges, women are educated in precisely the same manner as men are in men's colleges. The effect of such misguided education is that women are encouraged to develop aspirations which were designed exclusively to meet the needs of men.

Ashley Montagu understood nearly five decades ago that women were experiencing identity crises, and he attributed much of the confusion to the limitations of higher education. When women are educated to become like men and adopt men's values, then women will certainly learn to behave like men. As admirable a goal as it may be to establish a gender-neutral society, women continue to perform a function that is completely unique to women: they bear children who need to be cared for and reared.

Child-rearing is a serious endeavor that is integral to womanhood for most women. For this reason I agree wholeheartedly with Ashley Montagu (1967, 207) when he declares the following: "I put it down as an axiom that no woman with a husband and small children can hold a full-time job and be a good homemaker at one and the same time." Unfortunately, many women regard such sensible thinking as outdated and misguided chauvinism.

Women are now educated to do as men have done for generations: women are choosing to leave the care of home and children to someone other than themselves. As frequently as fathers in the past might have acknowledged their right to do as they pleased because they earned the family income, women are now invoking the same argument. Consequently, young children are being asked to forgo not only a father's availability but also a mother's.

There is a huge difference, however, between a father leaving the care of his children to his wife versus both parents leaving the care of their children to a nonrelative caregiver or an institution. Ultimately, the goal of modern living may be to eradicate the role of a mother in her child's life. This cannot be done, however, without causing great and perhaps irreparable harm to the well-being of children, their parents, and society at large.

The idea that the maternal role can be eliminated elucidates how unaware the general public is about human development and human relations. Simply stated, regardless of socioeconomic and educational backgrounds, many parents misunderstand the course of healthy human development. Moreover, modern education does not help women and men to understand much about children or their development. In fact, it appears that the more educated and the more financially successful parents are, the less they understand their children's needs.

Consider the case of a prominent lawyer who is described as follows:

> Molly Munger…is determined not to let her two children slow her down and finds she needs an outward focus to her life. She returned to work as a litigator within five weeks after the births of each of her two sons. She had intended to take three months off after her first son was born but ended up calling her boss and begging to return earlier. "All babies do is eat and sleep,"she says. "It was uninteresting to be around them. Their needs were easily met by others." Munger and her husband, also a lawyer, now employ two au pairs to care for their children in their Pasadena home. During the week Munger spends two hours each morning with the children. When she and her husband arrive home from work in Los Angeles their children are already asleep (Abramson and Franklin 1984, 194).

Molly Munger, a 1974 graduate of Harvard Law School, is like many contemporary parents in that she perceives the needs of her young babies to be unrelated to her. She assesses that her role as a mother is no different from that of any other caregiver in her babies' lives when she says, "Their needs were easily met by others."

RESPONSIVE MOTHERING

Indeed, many parents are inclined to think that a mother's role in her young child's life is neither unique nor special because anyone can supposedly feed a baby, change diapers and clothing, and keep the baby safe. The general idea is that hired help can easily do what a loving and caring mother does for her baby. For many parents, then, infant care revolves simply around satisfying a baby's physical needs.

A baby's needs, however, are markedly different from those of an adult. Consider, for instance, the dynamics surrounding a baby's hunger. An adult may eat when he feels hungry, or he can defer eating since he usually has sufficient stores of energy reserves in fat and muscle cells to stave off hunger. In contrast, a baby has no such reserves, and he needs to eat much more frequently in order to simply maintain a sense of satiety and nourish his quickly growing body. A baby's hunger is a real and forceful component of his existence that he cannot ignore through will.

A baby's needs are integrally related to his entire being, and the primary way in which he can communicate his needs is to cry aloud. Parents should try to imagine how difficult it is for a young baby to communicate in the absence of the ability to speak. An adult can understand how impaired communication becomes when he experiences a minor case of laryngitis. If another person is willing to understand the adult's gestures and hints, then communication might still be possible without speech. If, however, the other person is either unwilling or unable to try to understand what the adult is communicating, the adult's frustration will increase. One must imagine, then, how exasperating it must be for a baby when his cries are ignored by his caregivers.

Parents' decision to disregard their baby's cries is a culturally acquired parenting practice. There are societies in which young babies and children do not cry to the extraordinary extent that American and European babies do. For instance, anthropologist Meredith F. Small (1998, 154) cites a study of 160 Korean infants that "found no infants that could be classified as colicky, no clear crying peak at two months, and apparently no cluster of evening crying." The study notes that baby care in Korea, as compared to that in the U.S., entails a significantly greater amount of close physical contact and responsiveness. Thus, one-month-old Korean babies spend about two hours, or 8.3 percent of their time alone, versus one-month-old American babies who spend 67.5 percent of their time alone.

Clearly, the average American baby spends significantly more time alone than does his Korean counterpart. Additionally, Korean mothers respond to their babies' cries more quickly and consistently whereas American mothers tend to ignore much of their babies' crying. Whereas the initiation of a baby's cry appears to be universal, the parental response to a baby's cry is determined primarily by the culture in which the baby's parents have been reared.

One learns to parent from one's cultural upbringing, parents and siblings, extended family, friends, other parents, neighbors, acquaintances, books, magazines, newspapers, television, movies, daily experiences, and all else to which one has been and continues to be exposed. Everything one observes, learns, and absorbs from the environment becomes part of one's culture. Consequently, if present-day culture advocates certain child-rearing practices, one assumes that these practices exist for sound reasons.

Regrettably, current child-rearing practices may not be based upon wisdom or compassion but on expediency. Whatever is convenient for parents may be acceptable, even if the result is that young babies and children are reared with less than optimal care. Therefore, if babies cry and express their dissatisfaction, parents and substitute caregivers may follow the advice of child-rearing experts who claim that babies are not harmed by crying for prolonged periods of time.

Such a view of infant crying ignores the fact that the crying baby is a growing and developing individual. Meredith Small (1998, 155) offers a more helpful and insightful understanding of infant behavior:

> When an infant cries inconsolably for hours, when its tiny body arches in frustration, when its fists punch the air in anger, we see the clearest example of the clash between biology and culture. The baby is responding to an environment that has been culturally altered, and for which it has not been biologically adapted. And this is the trade-off. The infant is biologically adapted to expect the constant physical attachment and care within which the human infant evolved millions of years ago. But in some cultures, such as the industrialized countries of Europe and North America, parents are opting for a more independent relationship from their babies. They choose to place babies in cribs and car seats rather than carry them all the time, to feed babies in intervals rather than continuously, and to respond less quickly to infant distress. Although this style provides parents with some freedom from the demands of

> the infant, it also comes with a cost—a crying baby who is not biologically adapted to the cultural change.

It may be true that the majority of babies will survive despite the unpleasant or unhappy nature of their life circumstances. The direction of their human development, however, would be more positive and more humane if parents would choose to provide young babies and children with a more ideal environment in which to grow and develop.

CHOOSING TO BE A CHILD'S PRIMARY CAREGIVER

The logistics of staying home with one's baby can be difficult, particularly when parents incur significant financial obligations before the birth of their children. I know many working couples who purchased condominiums and houses in Los Angeles during a strong and costly real estate market boom in the late 1980s. Throughout the 1990s the obligation of meeting an expensive monthly mortgage forced many of my friends to join the legions of mothers of young children who work outside the home.

My situation was different since a combination of insufficient funds and my husband's pragmatism prevented us from buying a home. As much as I wanted to own a home, paying a monthly mortgage on my husband's income alone was impossible. We did, however, have the option of renting an apartment in a safe neighborhood, and I was able to stay home to rear our children. The restrictions of a limited income taught me the significance of frugality and avoiding debt.

Frugality is not a well-recognized virtue in our consumer-oriented society. It is now widely acknowledged that consumer spending constitutes two-thirds of the national Gross Domestic Product (GDP). President George W. Bush tried to bolster consumer spending further by endorsing major tax cuts worth billions of dollars during his first term in office. Additionally, when asked by citizens what they should do in response to the tragedy of September 11, 2001, President Bush advised them to shop. It is dispiriting that frugality and the saving of income are not encouraged since this is precisely what would enable more women to stay home with their young children.

Even though many mothers of young children wish they could stay home and not work outside the home, staying home is deemed to be financially impossible or impractical. The media report frequently that most mothers of young children work outside the home for financial reasons. Hence, if a mother can choose to stay home, then she is considered to be lucky since she can enjoy a luxury the majority of women cannot afford. In a way, a woman's decision to stay home with her young children is thought to be quaint and antiquated.

Invariably, a woman's decision to stay home invokes images of the 1950s suburban homemaker, but the reality is that few women today feel deep kinship toward homemakers of yore. I have a friend, for instance, who was a typical 1950s suburban housewife with a devoted husband and two children. Her husband insisted that she not work outside the home because he had been orphaned in early childhood; he wanted his children to be reared by their mother. In order to sustain their middle-class lifestyle, her husband held two or three jobs and worked long hours away from home. They lived for over forty years in the same small tract house in an affordable suburb of Los Angeles.

Like most stay-at-home mothers of her generation, my friend was an active member of her community. She spent many years as a volunteer and leader in her children's school PTA, Little League Baseball, Cub Scouts, Boy Scouts, and other community activities. Together with other mothers, they formed a cohesive group of women who enjoyed being stay-at-home mothers of Baby Boomers. These women's primary role was to care for home and family, and their active participation within their local communities was a significant secondary role.

I have another friend who also was a 1950s housewife. She is an intelligent woman who married right after high school and did not attend college. Her husband was a physician, and she learned a great deal about medicine from him. She could have pursued higher education at any time and become a physician herself. Instead, she opted to dedicate herself to her family, and to this day she spends the majority of her time fretting about her grown children and her grandchildren.

Although the responsibilities of homemaking and civic volunteerism were expected to last a lifetime, many homemakers learned that these activities were self-limiting. Children grew older, left home for college, and established their own families. As women aged, homemaking became a matter of housekeeping that required less work and could be performed efficiently perhaps by low-paid house cleaners. Grocery shopping and the need to cook were not nearly as imperative once children were no longer in the home. Also, opportunities to volunteer outside the home diminished since mothers generally worked in activities related mostly to their children's education and recreation. For many women, then, it was not a simple task to find outlets for their energy and intellect once the demands of homemaking and volunteerism waned.

Today, any woman who chooses to stay home with her children will face a similar situation: her children will mature and opportunities to volunteer for activities related to her children's education and recreation will decrease. In contrast to 1950s housewives, and thanks to the women's movement, women today have been better educated and trained to become capable and worthy employees or employers. Once child-rearing responsibilities ease, women can do a great deal because they are talented and have been educated to accomplish diverse goals. The conditions that may have bound women to the home indefinitely in the past, such as inferior education and limited work opportunities, are no longer as relevant or prevalent.

If anything, women are now facing the reverse situation: better education and social forces compel mothers to leave their young children far too soon. Whereas women were once tied to the home for too long, many women today are now almost not bound to the home at all. This trend in child-rearing has been occurring with the full approval of many men who think that women should be working outside the home in order to use their education, talents, and work experience to produce more family income.

In truth, there is a middle road that women today could choose in order to fulfill the needs of young children as well as their own. If the importance of the first five to six years of a child's life were to be established definitively, then perhaps the role of a mother would be more understandable to parents. However many years it may take, stay-at-home mothering will be a temporary situation and a mother's commitment to care for her young children will not forever bind her to the home.

In light of the approximately seventy-five year life span of the average American woman, a decade or more spent at home with one's children should not be overwhelming. Time passes quickly, and there is little reason to think that spending time at home as a mother is not as rewarding as time spent pursuing any other occupation. Stay-at-home mothering is invariably a time-consuming endeavor, but each woman will experience and value it in her unique way.

THE VALUE OF STAYING HOME

Although I could have earned a substantial income and enjoyed a higher standard of living as a working physician, I would not have been able to respond readily to my children's needs. For instance, although our daughter enjoyed an outstanding year of Kindergarten, she barely tolerated a miserable experience in the first grade at a new school: she cried every day for nearly three months. We finally pulled her out, and I home schooled her. We determined the following year that I should home school our son.

Fortunately, I was available to home school both children when they needed to leave the school system. Although our children could have endured their schooling experiences if we had chosen to do nothing, my presence at home provided us with an alternative that alleviated their distress and suffering. Staying home gave me the broad mandate to help my children when they needed me.

The cost of living is high, and one can readily understand why parents may think it is passé for a mother to stay home with her young children. Many women today give birth with the intention of returning to work fairly immediately since their employment offers income as well as work benefits like health insurance and a retirement plan. The U.S. government does little, if anything, to help women stay home to care for their young children.

The Swedish government, in comparison, provides long maternity and paternity leaves with stipends for mothers and fathers. Also, a Swedish mother's job is guaranteed for at least a year, and a return to part-time work is a viable option. In contrast, if American women wish to stay home with young babies, they need to have spouses who can provide a sufficient income and health insurance. If they are lucky and willing to accept help, parents can sometimes receive financial assistance from their own parents.

Since it costs money to do anything, practicing frugality has long been a way of life for our family. It can be simultaneously amusing and irritating for my adolescent son to realize how seriously our family takes the habit of frugality. For instance, when we go out to see a movie, we generally buy the largest tub of popcorn and share it among the four of us. I also bring our own bottles of water. Several months ago I had promised my son that we would not disturb his pleasure in seeing a movie at the theater. Unfortunately, our seating arrangement precluded any such assurance. We wound up passing popcorn to one another over his lap, and I cannot recall how many times he rolled his eyes with annoyance.

It makes sense that families should be encouraged to be frugal and direct their resources toward creating a more fulfilled family life. Living frugally requires discipline and self-control. Spending freely in the absence of sufficient income, on the contrary, reflects a lack of common sense and has the potential to create significant problems.

WOMEN AS CONSUMERS

The current state of the American economy was the topic of discussion on a September 27, 2004, *National Public Radio* broadcast on KCRW in Los Angeles. The panelists agreed that the U.S. economy is in poor shape because Americans tend to borrow and spend a large amount of money whereas they do not save enough money. As a country, the U.S. is getting into greater debt each year, and the panelists recommend that citizens and the government should borrow and spend less money.

Ironically, in the name of boosting the economy, modern society defies the logic of encouraging frugality. Instead, families are urged to spend more money. Thus, in recent decades, as women and children have become prime targets of the advertising industry, their spending has increased concordantly. This spending can keep increasing only as long as more women continue to work outside the home, even if it means leaving their young babies and children in the care of others. Since there are so many costs associated with working outside the home, there is little chance of increasing savings for the future. Thus, most of the money women earn is not saved but spent fairly quickly.

In the current economy, families do not need much encouragement to spend money. Unspoken rivalry in the past may have encouraged individuals to compete with their neighbors and friends or to "compete with the Joneses" by obtaining more or nicer things. This type of thinking has grown in magnitude such that everyone is supposed to procure a nice lifestyle. In a way, it seems egalitarian that any individual can purchase good quality merchandise and improve one's appearance and one's home. This illusion is perpetuated by the free market and the seemingly endless array of high-quality or good-quality items that can be bought at relatively low prices.

The December 12, 2004, issue of the *Los Angeles Times* features an article by Peter Gosselin entitled "The Poor Have More Things Today—Including Wild Income Swings." The article describes a hard working immigrant couple from El Salvador who were recently evicted from their long-time home. A front-page photograph of the family in their temporary home features their large color television set and computer. The text of the article reveals that the couple earn together approximately $18,000 per year (although they earned nearly double that prior to the downturn of the economy after September 2001), and they owe about $32,000 in credit card debts at a usurious rate of nearly 32 percent.

Approximately half of the credit card debt was incurred to pay for hospital bills associated with the births of the couple's two children in the U.S. The rest of the debt accumulated as a result of the couple's acquisition of many goods that reflected the purchasing power of their past income. The discrepancy between the couple's hard work, current insufficient income, enormous debt, and spending habits is discouraging. It is evident that many consumers no longer use common sense.

The banking conglomerates do not help consumers since they are interested only in generating greater profits. Thus, their policies tend to be cruel and unsympathetic toward the many consumers they attract through their advertisements. The offer of seemingly limitless credit to all sectors of the general public, including those with insufficient income, lures members of every demographic group possible to procure a lifestyle that revolves around active consumerism.

Consumerism is such a dominant force in modern society that the lifestyles of a significant percentage of American families today cannot be sustained without emphasizing work life. The spending habits of debt-laden consumers drive the American economy, and parents are a prime target for advertisers. In order to earn the income that the average family thinks it deserves to spend, however, family life is sacrificed significantly. It is a matter of course now that many families think they can enhance the quality of family life by spending more money. This may mean that parents are buying their children more toys and books, dining out more often with their children, or taking better family vacations.

To pay for all the things that are supposed to improve the quality of family life, nevertheless, increasing numbers of parents succumb to the domination of work life over home life. It is only a fortunate and small minority of citizens who earn excellent incomes and dividends from good savings and investment plans; they can afford to indulge in consumerism. The less fortunate majority may earn income that often needs to be supplemented by either increasing the number of hours they work or incurring more debt; these citizens cannot afford to consume too much, but they may do so anyway.

THE RISK OF BECOMING A MOTHER

It has long been politically incorrect to suggest that women can and should stay home to rear young children. As noble and significant as hands-on mothering is to the well-being of family, the pursuit of lifestyle and security is deemed to be an inevitable part of reality. As mentioned earlier, the modern era is not ideal for child-rearing.

In *The Price of Motherhood*, economics journalist Ann Crittenden argues that an American woman who becomes a mother will pay dearly for the rest of her life for making this single life decision. A woman might comprehend how becoming a mother will sidetrack her career, decrease her income, alter her social status, and diminish prospects for the social and political connections that often secure career advancement. Beyond these potential losses, however, Crittenden determines that motherhood in America is fraught with a risk few women consider prior to becoming mothers: the possibility of experiencing poverty.

Crittenden's book stresses the financial vulnerability that most American women risk today by becoming mothers. According to her book, women hazard a great deal in order to rear children since they undertake this responsibility with minimal compensation and without a financial or social safety net. She argues that women who perform the invaluable job of nurturing the next generation deserve, at a minimum, a financial safety net.

Crittenden proposes several measures that would better protect women who create and nurture society's next generation of citizens, workers, and taxpayers. She recommends that the tax burden on working women be eased by enabling them to file income tax returns independently of their spouses. She advocates giving mothers paid maternity leaves with guarantee of employment and the opportunity to return to work part-time without impairing career advancement opportunities. She suggests that the federal government sponsor nationwide day care centers that are modeled upon the high quality day care centers provided to American military personnel.

On the whole, Crittenden maintains that the family unit cannot perform the important task of child-rearing alone in the modern era. Crittenden reiterates often in her book that an American married woman with children is only a divorce away from poverty. The grim statistics and scenarios she describes in her book attest to the difficulty of rearing children in the U.S.

From Crittenden's perspective, it seems ludicrous to suggest that an ideal way of rearing children would include stay-at-home mothering, on demand and prolonged breastfeeding, and co-sleeping. All these activities require, at significant cost, a mother's presence in the home with her baby or young child. Despite Crittenden's reservations, however, it is more than possible for parents to defy divorce statistics and provide their children with maternal care.

Crittenden's book is important since it clarifies how costly it is for women to rear children today. Regardless of this reality, child-rearing is a responsibility that many parents undertake willingly and frequently without calculating only the financial costs involved. Undoubtedly, Crittenden would claim this position to be both naïve and impractical. She might be correct, but it does not mean that parents can no longer accomplish the goal of rearing their children in the nuclear family setting.

As mentioned earlier, even though the 1950s was not an ideal era for child-rearing, there was tacit and overt support for the prevalent and praiseworthy ethic of enabling women to stay home and rear children. In no way am I advocating a return to stay-at-home mothering under the same conditions as that of the 1950s. Times have changed significantly, and much of standard child-rearing advice of yore was questionable.

In that era, for example, bottle-feeding was declared to be superior to breast-feeding, and corporal punishment was the norm. Routinely, mothers were advised to distance themselves from their babies lest they become spoiled, and they were urged not to follow their intuition but to trust instead the authority of child-rearing experts. Despite these severe limitations of child-rearing practices in that era, however, many children benefited from receiving maternal care, even if that care happened to be tainted with some maternal resentment.

In stark contrast, stay-at-home mothering today has lost so much value and respect that many people dismiss outright the need for maternal care. Parents are informed routinely that it is impossible to rear young children on one income alone. In an April 29, 2001, article entitled "Bringing Down Baby" in the *Los Angeles Times,* Peggy Orenstein (who was not then a mother) writes the following in support of day care: "It is pathetic, in the year 2001, to have to remind people that two incomes are necessary for basic survival in most families.... Day care, which now serves 13 million children, is here to stay. Working mothers are here to stay...If anything is harmful to children, it's the false debate over whether mothers should stay home..." The de facto way in which Orenstein writes belies the ability of parents to adjust their lifestyles and priorities in order to permit a mother to stay home with her children.

THE COST OF STAYING HOME

It might not be easy, but there are many couples who make significant sacrifices in order to permit mothers to stay home with young children. For instance, I have a friend who stayed home full-time to rear her two daughters. Her husband was a biology instructor and she held a Master's degree in linguistics. The family lived on a small income, rented a modest apartment, and rarely drove their old Toyota. Their dinnerware consisted of different pieces of earthenware that their children had made at the local recreation center. They managed because they had the conviction that breastfeeding and maternal care were best for their young children.

It is possible for families to rear children on one income irrespective of what the pundits may write. Two parents who are committed to one another and their children can make stay-at-home mothering a practical aspect of family life. Such commitment, regardless of what the costs may be, is sadly thought to be exceptional since the modern family unit is far from stable.

Crittenden, for instance, describes couples whose marriages disintegrate even when young children are involved. She portrays callous men who divorce their wives despite knowing that their former wives and their children will experience decreased income or even poverty. In many cases of divorce, it is women who sacrifice careers and income in order to rear children. In some situations, women support their husbands through professional schooling, help secure their husbands' professions, and then wind up in unpredictable financial situations after their husbands divorce them.

These men lack humanity. If a man falls in love with another woman, or he decides his marriage cannot be salvaged, his minimal responsibility is to make sure that his former wife and children are financially secure. This is the least reassurance a man can give his former wife, a person he presumably loved at some point.

From this perspective, men who plan to divorce their wives should behave as admirably as does Frank Algernon Cowperwood, the protagonist of Theodore Dreiser's novel *The Financier*. This novel was written over a century ago, but its accurate portrayal of a failed marriage is still relevant today. Frank Cowperwood is a married man who, after falling in love with a younger woman, seeks to extricate himself from his first marriage.

Dreiser offers a sympathetic portrait of Frank as a passionate but responsible man. Although Frank is in love with another woman, he must take into consideration the welfare of Lillian and their children. Fortunately for Lillian, Frank must be reasonable and generous because she has to agree to grant him a divorce. When her financial outlook improves alongside his business successes, the two work out an amicable divorce agreement. The divorce situation faced by the fictional Lillian Cowperwood does not, unfortunately, resemble the much less favorable divorce situations many women experience in the modern era.

Crittenden asserts that women who face divorce are clearly at a disadvantage since the majority of lawmakers and judges are biased against reducing a man's income in order to support his ex-wife and children. Additionally, a man's second spouse can often be unsympathetic to the plight of the first wife and her children; she may even discourage her spouse from offering support for the ex-wife. Thus, a woman who has dedicated herself to child-rearing either on a full-time or part-time basis is unlikely to maintain a lifestyle comparable to that which she had before her divorce. From this perspective, Crittenden's book is significant since it emphasizes the need for every woman to become financially astute before she contemplates marriage and motherhood.

In general, there are no legal safeguards that enable women to gain access to their husbands' income. If the husband is the primary breadwinner, as is usually the case when women stay home to care for their children, the husband apparently has the right to spend his income as he pleases whereas his spouse does not. Since the sharing of earned income is often done at the discretion of the husband, it would be best for women to comprehend how to secure their financial well-being prior to marrying.

Although Crittenden's intention may be to portray the reality of modern mothering, she makes it appear as if stay-at-home mothering is completely impractical. She even declares that the American Academy of Pediatrics' guideline for infants to be breastfed for at least the first twelve months of life is a "sick joke." Crittenden describes breastfeeding as an elitist activity that only well-educated and financially well-off women can afford.

In many ways, the culture of breastfeeding today does exist primarily in the moneyed and educated sectors of the American population although there may be ethnic groups in which breastfeeding is the norm and supported by family and community. The widespread availability and advertisement of infant formula in the United States, however, influence many immigrants to use infant formula even though they would have routinely breastfed in their country of origin. For example, in the late 1980s a friend of mine worked in a Los Angeles birthing clinic in which nearly all Hispanic women breastfed their newborns. In contrast, if one looks about in public arenas today, the majority of Hispanic babies appear to be bottle-fed with infant formula.

The current culture of breastfeeding in the U.S. is centered upon women who have the financial means and the educational background to seek alternatives to conventional infant and child care. Accordingly, the cost of obtaining sound information about breastfeeding may be prohibitively high. For instance, a local Los Angeles pediatrician is an outspoken advocate of prolonged breastfeeding who happens to charge high fees for his consultations. Those who are financially well off or well-educated can afford or are willing to pay for this pediatrician's care.

Fortunately for this pediatrician's patients, he speaks frankly about the superiority of breastfeeding and provides parents with the auxiliary support to succeed with breastfeeding. Every mother who chooses to breastfeed in his medical practice receives a home visit by a lactation consultant within days of the baby's birth to evaluate the progress of breastfeeding. Every baby receives a check-up at two weeks of age to assure his well-being. Naturally, all of this support requires financial resources that many women do not possess.

Crittenden may be correct in asserting that the culture of breastfeeding in the United States is, in many ways, restricted to a relatively small population of highly educated mothers. It is also within this population group that babies are breastfed longer. As discussed earlier, however, it was wealthy and educated women at the turn of the twentieth century who engendered the demise of breastfeeding by acceding to the authority of physicians and the science of infant feeding. It is ironic and just that educated women today are creating the trend that will direct women back toward the meaningful and important art of breastfeeding.

The case for staying home may appear to be impractical if one assumes that half of marriages fail, but families are capable of creating a cohesive unit that prioritizes the well-being of children and their mothers. Parents need to incorporate the cost of stay-at-home mothering into their budgets prior to having children. In this way, parents can judge for themselves whether or not the cost of having a mother care directly for their children can be managed. This is a decision that must be undertaken by both parents. Without the cooperation of the father, it is highly unlikely that a mother can continue to stay home with her child. Also, a father certainly has to be interested enough in his family to partake fully in his role as a family breadwinner.

The family situation in which the father is the sole breadwinner is not a throwback to the Dark Ages, as some feminists would argue. Rather, it is a healthy family situation in which the father is wise, compassionate, and humane, particularly if he upholds monogamy and cherishes his wife with love and appreciation. Every woman should be lucky enough to have such a spouse, and every baby should be fortunate enough to have such a father.

In the final analysis, it is probable that children who have been reared humanely and with unconditional love will mature into healthy and loving men and women. These men and women can nurture another generation of caring children who will also mature into loving and humane adults. Dedication to family and community is a learned behavior that is transmitted from generation to generation. Those who value motherhood learn how to respect motherhood at some point in their own lives. On the other hand, there are far too many people who do not learn why they should respect motherhood.

12

A MOTHER'S IDENTITY

"ONLY A MOTHER"

By abdicating employment outside the home in order to care for her children, a woman may earn the distinction of being "only a mother." The disdain for women who stay home is often overt. Most stay-at-home mothers encounter unpleasant remarks such as the following: "What do you do all day?"; "When are you returning to work?"; "Oh, you're not returning to work?"; "Don't you get bored?"; "Don't you miss your career?"; "Don't you miss the intellectual stimulation of seeing anyone other than your baby?"; "Aren't you wasting your education?"; and "Don't you feel like you're not achieving or doing anything?" It is fairly easy to notice the prejudice in these pejorative questions.

I have encountered these questions as well as other inquiries and criticisms over the years, but there are many women who have been subjected to disrespectful contempt and disdain. For example, I know mothers who have met men and women who walked away from them with the attitude that they could not be bothered to speak with someone who was "only a mother." A friend's husband indicates that this type of dismissive behavior may occur because some men and women are either simply uncomfortable with the notion of mothers staying home or they might feel guilty because they are not providing their own children with similar care. This is probably true, but it offers little consolation for sensible and intelligent women who are demeaned because they stay home to rear their children.

For the past few decades, women have been growing up with the idea that becoming a mother is a choice or a desire whereas working outside the home is a necessity. Women learn that motherhood is not a full-time occupation but a slight detour along the path of life that is not supposed to affect one's lifestyle significantly. Accordingly, short maternity leaves and a return to work outside the home soon after a baby's birth have become the norm in the U.S.

One has to wonder how mothering lost its appeal as a worthwhile occupation, so much so that millions of women choose not to care for their own children today. It is not even that most mothers want to leave their children behind in order to work. Consistently, most women polled express their preference to stay home with their young children. For instance, in a 2000 poll performed by Youth Intelligence, a Manhattan-based market research firm, 68 percent of women between the ages of 18 and 34 say that "they would prefer to stay at home and raise their children to working outside the home" (Mokros 2002). Despite many polls that reveal the same findings, it is widely understood that the majority of mothers will no longer care directly for their own children.

Moreover, the fact that most women will not earn much money does not appear to deter women from returning to work outside the home. The majority of women work outside the home as teachers, administrators, secretaries, assistants, store clerks, sales clerks, vocational nurses, day care workers, hospital aides, medical technicians, factory workers, civil employees, domestic cleaners, and so forth. Only a minority of women are employed in higher paying and more prestigious professions such as law, medicine, business, accounting, academia, journalism, publishing, and entertainment. In truth, there is a huge discrepancy in compensation that is given to women for their various occupations outside the home. Even so, the overwhelming domination of work life over home life almost guarantees that the majority of women with young children at home will continue to work outside the home.

Currently, more than 79 percent of women with school-aged children work outside the home (Nightingale and Fix 2004). When women have so many obligations to work outside the home, fewer have the time and energy to create a meaningful home life. Although a significant aspect of being "only a mother" is to develop and maintain a consequential home life, such work is not truly appreciated. This may not be a new phenomenon, but a consequence of ignoring home life is that the quality of home life is deteriorating for many families.

Susan Cheever (1995, 86), in the *New Yorker* article cited earlier about deprived children, offers a description of the home in which the nanny, Dominique, works: "It's a modern apartment, with lots of light, but it's crowded with furniture and unopened mover's boxes are piled in one corner. The kitchen counters are overflowing with dishes, and the cabinets are filled with paper plates and appliances that are still in bubble wrap. When Dominique took this job, six months ago, Suzanne explained that they had just moved in. Later, Dominique found out that they had 'just moved in' in 1992." The couple is so busy with work outside the home that they have not yet unpacked boxes even though they moved into their apartment more than two years earlier.

This family is fortunate that a paid helper is willing and able to do the work that the mother apparently has neither the time nor interest to do. From Cheever's description, Dominique does a great deal to improve the quality of the children's home life. There are nevertheless serious limitations as to what a substitute caregiver can offer young children, especially when there is an unsettled and chaotic atmosphere to the home situation. Such a lifestyle, however, may be the inevitable consequence of women's insistence that they have more important things to do than the work of homemaking and being "only a mother."

FROM SELF-SUFFICIENCY TO DEPENDENCY

For well over a century, women have been grappling with the meaning of their role in home life and work life. The late historian and social critic Christopher Lasch notes that many women had already become dissatisfied with the roles they played in family life by the turn of the twentieth century. In *Haven in a Heartless World: The Family Besieged*, Lasch offers a compelling history of the various factors that affected the American family and, in particular, women.

Lasch emphasizes that the Industrial Revolution during the nineteenth century had a far greater and more negative impact upon home life and family life than is generally appreciated. Industrialization affected women's productivity immensely and engendered new questions about the role of women in the home. Prior to industrialization, the home was a veritable center of production since there were few goods and services that families needed to purchase.

The work done in the home was invaluable since women did numerous chores that made most families nearly self-sufficient. Women gardened, canned fruits and vegetables, cooked and baked, sewed and mended clothing, washed and ironed clothing, cleaned house, reared children, and did all else to maintain the well-being of those in their homes. The advent of canned and processed food, home appliances, manufactured clothing, and prefabricated furniture and household goods, however, made a great deal of women's work obsolete.

Christopher Lasch (1977, 9) offers the following astute observation: "Industry had invaded the family, stripped it of its productive functions." Although women still had a great deal of work to do in the home, it was not nearly of the magnitude that countless generations of women had performed before. Consequently, confusion arose among different factions of women as to what role women should be playing in the home and in society.

While feminists advocated that women should no longer be self-sacrificing or of service to others, critics of feminists sought to ennoble women's domestic roles. Lasch (1977, 10) notes that "critics of feminism began to argue that motherhood and housewifery themselves constituted satisfying 'careers,' which required special training in 'homemaking,' 'domestic science,' and 'home economics.' The invention of such terms expressed an attempt to dignify housework by raising it to the level of a profession.... Ironically, the rationalization of housework rendered the housewife more dependent than ever on the help of outside experts." Evidently, the attempt to validate the importance of domestic work, which included foremost the responsibility of child-rearing, was successful.

Unfortunately, it was not women's wisdom and abilities that were exalted. Instead, psychologists, social workers, physicians, and educators became professional consultants to whom women became obliged for child-rearing guidance. Paradoxically, these professionals gleaned their knowledge and wisdom from mothers and then declared themselves to be more knowledgeable about mothering than mothers themselves.

Over a short span of time, women became beholden not only to domestic science experts for housekeeping advice but also to hosts of new experts for child-rearing advice. The independent woman who controlled and managed a household efficiently was now a woman who no longer had sufficient wisdom or knowledge to rear her own children. The new homemaker was no longer self-reliant: she instead relied on the advice of a slew of therapists and experts who were armed with dogma that was masked as scientific progress.

Lasch refers to this entire process of stripping parents, particularly mothers, of parental authority and undermining their wisdom and knowledge as the "proletarization of parenthood." Whereas families had generally been autonomous, parents were suddenly in need of expert advice from educators and social workers. There was, in fact, so little confidence in the family unit that these experts sought to improve the quality of family life by offering parent education programs, marriage counseling, and psychiatric social work. The general idea was that parents alone could no longer accomplish the important task of rearing children without a bureaucracy of therapists and academicians who would oversee parental functions.

It is unnerving to learn that the general assumption made by leading sociologists a century ago was that society itself would eventually take the place of the family. Lasch (1977, 13) points out that "the family did not simply evolve in response to social and economic influences; it was deliberately transformed by the intervention of planners and policymakers." Long ago, then, schools and social welfare agencies were given a great deal of power and control over families.

Lasch describes how workers in the "helping professions," which included educators, psychiatrists, social workers, and penologists, insisted that they were acting as doctors in a sick society. Lasch (1977, 18) notes that these forces of "society in the guise of a 'nurturing mother' invaded the family, the stronghold of those private rights, and took over many of its functions." Over a matter of mere decades, the autonomy of family life was dismantled by impersonal bureaucrats who usurped parental authority and demeaned summarily a woman's unique role in family life.

Meanwhile, feminists argued that if the family could be stripped of its productive function by industrialization, then everything else associated with family life, including child-rearing, recreation, and housework, could also be taken over by outside agencies. This would enable women to "follow their work out of the home" and not be confined to the family as parasites and unproductive "consumers upon the state" (Lasch 1977, 9). By emphasizing the primacy of getting women paid for working outside the home and not inside the home, however, feminists aligned themselves with the economic forces that were insidiously and successfully undermining the meaning of family life. Far from being radical and improving the status of women, the feminist movement succeeded primarily in further devaluing family life.

THE FEMINIST AGENDA

For many years feminists have lobbied for women's right to work outside the home, irrespective of the presence of young children in the home. Assuredly, the women's movement has enhanced women's access to equal education and improved work opportunities for the good of girls, women, and society. The same movement has also, however, played a significant role in diminishing the value of women's work in the home.

In general, despite or perhaps because of the enormity of the job of mothering, it is increasingly becoming work that falls into the hands of hired help. According to data from the U.S. Department of Labor (2005), "the median hourly earnings of wage and salary childcare workers were $7.86 in 2002, with the middle 50 percent earning between $6.66 and $9.65." The department states that child care workers "play an important role in a child's development by caring for the child when parents are at work or away for other reasons."

Better educated child care workers receive higher wages, but the converse is true as well. Additionally, there is a high turnover rate among child care workers, most of whom are generally paid "very low wages" with varied or no benefits. There are even some workers who are kept as indentured servants to do housekeeping and child-rearing. Irrespective of the vast amount of work that mothering and homemaking entail, most hired helpers are paid poorly.

The low value that is placed upon the care provided by child care workers reflects, in many ways, the view of some feminists. As far as they are concerned, educated and employable women who choose to stay home with their children are not much different from indentured servants. In a sense, there may be some validity to such a view. After all, many women who stay home are paid nothing at all even though they are on call for their children twenty-four hours per day, seven days a week. In truth, no professional would tolerate working under conditions comparable to those faced by mothers daily.

For instance, it would be difficult to find a physician or attorney who would provide for free the kind of attention and care to patients or clients that a mother gives her child. Although a mother pays even more attention to her children than does a physician to a patient or a lawyer to a client, a mother does not get paid whereas a physician or attorney can charge hundreds of dollars per hour. In spite of the enormous responsibilities of stay-at-home mothering, there is no remuneration, and a job well done is generally disregarded.

In many ways, mothering is taken for granted as something that will be accomplished regardless of how little contact a baby or child has with her mother. The adage "Once a mother, always a mother" assures many women of the biological bond that guarantees a woman's identity as mother to her child. Even as women work long hours outside the home, they trust that their motherhood should not be questioned, and it usually is not. Thus, in the case of an emergency, a child's mother is often contacted first even when a stay-at-home father is the child's primary caregiver. Most women are only too willing to respond to these calls because they are genuinely concerned about the well-being of their children.

Some feminists, however, disdain a mother's attachment to her child, and they deny rigorously the uniqueness of the mother-infant bond. They propose that a child should be attached equally to her caregivers, be it her father, mother, or any other provider of care. Their position is that if there is a unique mother-infant bond, then there should be a similarly special father-infant bond. In other words, the responsibility of child-rearing cannot be relegated to only the baby's mother since this is chauvinistic and unfair. In the supposedly enlightened modern era, the wisdom of the feminist agenda is that women should return to work outside the home and disregard the needs of their babies.

EVALUATING THE FEMINIST MOVEMENT

It is important and relevant to question how beneficial the feminist movement has been for family life. The majority of mothers with young infants are now in the workforce, which means that the majority of infants no longer receive maternal care. One can surely excuse and applaud the mothers who are performing unique and incomparable service to all of society by working outside the home.

A good example of such a capable and industrious mother is Marie Curie, the Nobel Prize-winning scientist. She was truly exceptional since she was able to contribute enormously to the advance of science while she managed to maintain a healthy and loving family life. Her daughter, Eve Curie, wrote *Madame Curie: A Biography*, which is a moving account of her mother's life.

It is improbable, however, that the greater majority of women can or will be able to make outstanding and invaluable contributions to society as did Marie Curie. This is not to proffer either prejudice against or discouragement to the many women who are participating actively in the work world. Rather, it is meant to draw attention to the incomparable importance of a woman's contributions to humanity by providing her child with unique maternal care. As significant and productive as work outside the home is, so is the priceless work that is done in the home that permits a child to mature and grow into a humane being.

In truth, no one can or should cast doubt on the value of any individual's occupation, including stay-at-home mothering. As it stands, the majority of women do not perceive mothering to be work that they necessarily need to perform. Women are now emphasizing work life over family life and child-rearing, just as men have been doing for many generations. As more and more parents work long hours outside the home, many children are placed in some form of organized care, or they are simply left unattended.

As a result, a disproportionate number of infants and young children are placed in day care and organized pre-school activities. Similarly, school-aged children spend longer hours in school, and many attend before-school and after-school child care facilities. Meanwhile, many pre-teens and teenagers spend more time home alone and unsupervised after school.

Some may contend that this is the reality of modern life since economics drives such changes in family life. There may be elements of truth in such a view, but it should be noted that the widespread neglect of family life and home life is astounding. Christopher Lasch (1977, xxi) offers the astute observation that "social change does not occur automatically but requires active human intervention." Many women may no longer care directly for their own young children in the twenty-first century, but this is solely because actions by men and women have driven such a societal trend.

THE IMPORTANCE OF MOTHERING

It is unfortunate that hands-on mothering is thought of as a relic of a bygone era since mothering will always be relevant to human existence. The truth is that there would be no humanity without women who bear children. This is not to say that women must bear children. Obviously, there are many women who lead fulfilling lives without bearing children. Even childless women, though, are not averse to expressing maternal behavior. For instance, I have an accomplished friend who has dedicated her life to academia, and she is content to think of her students as her children.

Maternal behavior is a source of pride for many women. For ages and ages, mothers were probably accorded due respect and appreciation. In recent years, however, it has become politically incorrect to recognize the importance of hands-on mothering. Concomitantly, the voices of discontented women who do not appreciate the value of mothering have become loud and influential.

In the meantime, life revolves around mothering in nearly every aspect of nature. All the technological and scientific advances of recent decades cannot ignore the fact that human beings are nurtured in and are borne from their mothers' wombs. Granted, there may be some confusion in the modern era since surrogate mothers and artificial reproductive methods have muddled the normal biological view of motherhood. Suffice it to say that the human newborn still needs to develop in and emerge from a woman's womb. For the majority of children, no one is as important as the mother who gave birth to her.

Life is nurtured with mothering, whether or not this fact is acknowledged. Simply stated, consistent and loving mothering is the basis for healthy human existence. Although it is encouraging that caregivers other than biological mothers can nurture babies and children, it must be acknowledged that successful surrogate caregiving is modeled upon loving and caring maternal behavior.

Surrogate care is important since there will always be babies and children who cannot be cared for by their biological mothers. Over the long span of human existence, however, most women were able to nurture their own children. The trend in modern culture, unfortunately, veers in the opposite direction since women are blatantly discouraged from mothering their own children.

Instead of acknowledging the importance of mothering, modern culture demands that parents look at every aspect of a child's care as consumption. A parent's time is measured carefully so that a baby is permitted to spend some time with his mother after she returns home from work. A baby may use a certain number of diapers and bottles of infant formula each day, so a weekly trip to the grocery store should provide an adequate supply. A baby must take naps at specified times of the day for a consistent amount of time. A baby needs a baby-sitter for at least nine hours per day, so the parents need to consider procuring the help of a relative, hiring a nanny, or perhaps using a day care center. These are some of the ways in which a child's care is quantified, but the overall effect is to dehumanize the task of mothering.

In general, mothering cannot be approached as a job that is measured primarily by efficiency. One cannot specify exactly how much time and effort are needed to help nurture the healthy development of a child. Also, mothering is an activity that will not necessarily guarantee a good outcome. Regardless of the sincerity and quality of parental efforts, some children will stray and become troubled individuals. Such variability in outcome is, however, no excuse for women to avoid undertaking and bearing the responsibility of mothering. If anything, it becomes that much more imperative to take the task of mothering seriously. Ultimately, consistent and loving mothering will benefit healthy child development immeasurably because so much of human development occurs subtly and inconspicuously.

Consider, for example, the meaningful ability of a healthy human being to be alone. Although one enjoys and learns the rudiments of healthy social interaction in the presence of loving family members and friends, one invariably needs to spend a great deal of time alone. Therefore, one needs to learn how to live in a healthy and fulfilling manner when one is alone just as much as one needs to learn how to live sociably with others.

Sadly, there are many examples of how incapable human beings are of creating value and living in peace alone. For instance, within the last year an upsurge in the production of opium in Afghanistan has resulted in the widespread distribution of potent heroin all over the world. A November 29, 2004, article by Jeffrey Fleishman in the *Los Angeles Times* reveals how the rampant use of heroin is affecting countless young adults in Oslo, Norway, a model welfare state. The article quotes an eighteen-year-old girl: "'I try to quit,' she said, her face pale in the autumn half-light. 'I get depressed, and I run away inside myself.'" This young woman has no idea how to live in peace by herself, for she did not develop the capacity to be alone in a healthy manner as a young child.

What enables a child to develop into a healthy adult who can live alone is the constancy of being around a loving and available caregiver. In an intriguing discussion of the importance of a mother's presence in a child's life, psychiatrist Anthony Storr cites the work of psychiatrist John Bowlby and psychoanalyst Donald Winnicott. Bowlby played a significant role in clarifying the consequences of maternal deprivation in English children over the course of a long career. He theorized the importance of attachment and asserted that a child becomes secure by attaching herself to her primary caregiver, which is ideally the child's mother.

In the secure presence of her mother, the child develops the capacity to be alone because she does not need to feel anxious about her mother's possible departure. In other words, the secure child will mature into an adult who can feel secure alone. Winnicott took attachment theory further and suggested that the capacity to be alone is related to an individual's ability to comprehend her own needs and true feelings.

Winnicott posited that an individual can discover what she wants or needs only after she develops the capacity to be alone first in the presence of her mother and then later without her mother. Storr (1988, 21) elaborates further: "The capacity to be alone thus becomes linked with self-discovery and self-realization; with becoming aware of one's deepest needs, feelings, and impulses." It is in the presence of a loving and available caregiver, ideally the mother, that a child develops the ability to comprehend her true self and learn what it is that she feels and needs.

The heroin addict cited earlier, in contrast, is unaware of her needs, feelings, or impulses. She is still searching to find herself, as are countless youngsters and adults all over the world who succumb to drug addiction and substance abuse. There is little doubt that there are far too many individuals who are as clueless as this young woman is. They are equally unaware of and seemingly incapable of knowing how to live productively and creatively on their own. From this perspective, it cannot be emphasized enough that consistent and loving mothering enables children to develop their true identities.

THE LUXURY OF MOTHERING

Transcending all strata of society, women can enjoy mothering at their own risk. Among the poor, mothering is a luxury not even welfare recipients may be permitted to experience. This means, of course, that indigent mothers will continue to have babies, but it is unlikely that they can actually care for their babies. Among the middle-class, women may reject stay-at-home mothering because the maintenance of careers and the procurement of a certain standard of living have gained primacy. Among the wealthy, mothering may actually become a pastime that gets squeezed in between social and charitable engagements, as well as commitments to self-improvement activities like prolonged gym workouts and beauty treatments. In other words, although women may bear babies, they may not necessarily do the work of mothering.

Over the past several decades, women have been taught to pursue higher education and earn educational degrees in order to gain meaningful and remunerative employment outside the home. Higher education, as discussed earlier, does not address the issues of child-rearing and mothering. Instead, the emphasis of modern education is to steer women away from home life and toward the big expanse of the work world. Such education has been highly influential. As much as men may have avoided the physical labor of child-rearing in the past, more women are now doing exactly the same thing.

What is intriguing is how a cultural mind-set can influence women strongly enough to make them ignore fundamental biology. This is not to argue that work outside the home is not an option for all women since more than half of mothers of children under the age of one are in the workforce. It is imperative to remember, though, that an option is a choice that an individual can make. Unfortunately, women today are almost told de facto that they cannot stay home with their young children.

A half century ago, women were expected to stay home, and now women are expected to stay in the workforce and outside the home. It is a small but powerful and vocal minority of women that advises legions of women that their presence in the lives of their babies and children is insignificant. Do women trust, however, that it is beneficial and healthy to withhold their physical presence from their children's lives? In the near future, it will become evident that women from the 1980s onward were pressured inordinately to work outside the home and acknowledge mothering as not being work at all.

13

FAMILY LIFE

FAMILY LIFE VERSUS WORK LIFE

At the turn of the twentieth century, the bureaucratic forces of medicine, sociology, and education worked together to undermine the autonomy of families. Although women had always performed vital functions within the home throughout history, the advent of experts in nearly every aspect of domestic life forced women to abdicate not only their independence but also their self-respect. As a natural consequence of having lost their autonomy, growing numbers of women became dissatisfied with being homemakers. As maternal wisdom and intuition were thrown by the wayside and the science of child-rearing turned mothers into mere consumers of expert advice, it became demoralizing to be only a mother and homemaker.

Over the past century, a different kind of woman began taking the place of the knowledgeable and independent homemaker who took pride in rearing her children and managing her household. A good, if not typical, example of this different kind of woman was Eleanor Roosevelt. Born into wealth as a homely child of stunningly attractive parents, Eleanor Roosevelt had a sad childhood. Eleanor Roosevelt experienced terrible and purposeful neglect from her gorgeous mother while her doting father, an alcoholic, was frequently absent from the home. Both parents died when she was young. Later, after marrying Franklin Delano Roosevelt (FDR), Eleanor was dominated by her mother-in-law, Sara Roosevelt, who actively encouraged her grandchildren to refer to her, not Eleanor, as their mother.

In *No Ordinary Time: Franklin and Eleanor Roosevelt: The Home Front in World War II*, the historian Doris Kearns Goodwin (1995, 97–98) relays how profoundly insecure Eleanor Roosevelt felt as a mother: "Forced to remain at home while her husband went to work, Eleanor found her old insecurities returning. So painful was the memory of her own tormented childhood that she approached the task of mothering with little joy.... It was only after her last child was born...that Eleanor found her identity. Free to define a new role for herself beyond her family, she poured all her pent-up energies into a variety of reformist organizations..." For various reasons, Eleanor Roosevelt did not enjoy mothering and homemaking whereas she eventually found great fulfillment in working outside the home.

During the World War II era, Mrs. Roosevelt traveled across the country and updated her husband on the condition of American citizens. This was a role that Goodwin describes as being one that Mrs. Roosevelt took great pride in because it gave her a chance to tell her husband about the problems that ordinary citizens faced in their daily lives. She traveled extensively at a time when the country needed to mobilize a huge workforce that could accommodate an expansive demand for wartime products such as airplanes, tanks, ships, submarines, and guns. With enormous contingents of men having been drafted into the armed services, there was a shortage of manpower in factories. One effective solution was to simply increase the number of women in the workforce.

In the 1930s and the 1940s, Eleanor Roosevelt was instrumental in supporting the entry of increased numbers of women into the workforce. Goodwin (369) describes how Mrs. Roosevelt reveled in hearing that women were contributing greatly to the wartime effort: "Eleanor took special pleasure in hearing that women were 'doing a swell job, better than they (supervisors) expected.'" As the war years continued and the need for workers increased, greater numbers of women, including mothers of young children, were drawn out of the home and into the workforce: by 1942 there were 19 million women in the workforce.

Mrs. Roosevelt lobbied energetically for women's participation in the workforce. She also had deep compassion for women who lost their jobs after the war ended. Goodwin describes how Mrs. Roosevelt listened with pride as women proclaimed their inability to return to homemaking after having encountered the wonder of operating lathes.

Women who worked at the factories and plants experienced the camaraderie, sense of accomplishment and usefulness, and income production that often accompany employment outside the home. The historian William Chafe (Goodwin 1995, 624) writes that the war effected change in women's lives as nothing else could: "Work had proved liberating and once a new consciousness had been formed, there was no going back." Increasingly, the value of homemaking was being challenged and questioned by growing numbers of women.

By the mid-1940s it was hard to argue that homemaking was such an incredible occupation in and of itself. Most homemakers were no longer authoritative and knowledgeable women who could manage their homes independently and resourcefully. Several decades had already passed since the advent of the experts who claimed to know more about child-rearing and homemaking than did the women who bore the children and took care of the home.

Child-rearing had become a science about which experts were espousing their views, and mothers were as intimidated as the experts expected them to be. Trusting that the answers to their domestic problems lay outside of their intuition and experience, women sought and paid for the advice of experts. In many ways women had been relieved of the significant and demanding responsibility of maintaining autonomy over family life.

At the same time, however, women were not relieved of the overall burden of bearing responsibility for the well-being of their families. This odd combination of disempowering women while still keeping them liable for the welfare of their families was disconcerting. It is no wonder that more women were finding child-rearing and homemaking to be tiresome, unproductive, and uninspiring.

In light of the conditions of homemaking in her day, one cannot blame an educated and intelligent woman like Mrs. Roosevelt for her disenchantment with homemaking and the duties of being a wife. She could not oblige her husband by serving him tea, sitting by his side as he sorted through his extensive stamp collection, or listening to his stories every day whereas his cousins and close women friends took great pleasure in these activities. Mrs. Roosevelt, instead, delighted in sharing with her husband her thoughts about the plight of working women who needed day care facilities for their children or the poor wages non-unionized workers received. The opportunity to engage her husband in discussions about numerous social issues brought her joy that homemaking did not.

Nevertheless, as intellectual and politically active as Mrs. Roosevelt was, she still had a definitive need to love and be loved, as do all human beings. According to Goodwin, Mrs. Roosevelt was particularly close to one young friend, Joe Lash, and she made great efforts both to see him and spend time with him. Her interest in family life might have been limited, but this did not mean that Mrs. Roosevelt did not seek love and affection from elsewhere. Invariably, human beings still hope to find the love that family life normally provides. Mrs. Roosevelt, the ultimate champion of work life over family life, was still a human being who needed to love and be loved.

Mrs. Roosevelt was obviously human, but the legacy she has left in her wake lacks humanity. The primacy of work life over family life is now the norm. With more than half of women with children under the age of one year in the workforce, women today embrace work life and set aside home life, much as Mrs. Roosevelt and her friends envisioned women should.

ESCAPE FROM FAMILY LIFE

Eleanor Roosevelt had already been a homemaker for many years before she dedicated her life to work outside the home. Goodwin (97) quotes Mrs. Roosevelt as having said, "For ten years I was always just getting over having a baby or about to have another one, and so my occupations were considerably restricted." According to Goodwin (97), Mrs. Roosevelt had expected to lead a fulfilling life with her husband, having "traded the chance for deeper involvement in social work for the hope of finding happiness as a wife and mother."

Unfortunately, Mrs. Roosevelt experienced a life-altering event: she was devastated by her husband's affair with the aristocratic beauty, Lucy Mercer. Although Mrs. Roosevelt had put her family life before her own career aspirations, her husband's affair changed everything. His infidelity paved the way for Mrs. Roosevelt to discover her identity outside of her family life.

A confluence of other factors, including the fact that Mrs. Roosevelt's children were no longer babies and that her mother-in-law interfered unduly in her domestic life, enabled her to cultivate her identity away from her family life and affix it instead to her work life. When Mrs. Roosevelt was in her mid-thirties, she began working for the League of Women Voters, which is where she met intelligent, articulate, hard-working, ambitious, and independent women. With the encouragement of these women, Mrs. Roosevelt cultivated her talents to become a greatly respected writer, orator, and social advocate.

Historian Doris Kearns Goodwin (208) remarks that when Mrs. Roosevelt first came into contact with the women at the League of Women Voters, she conceded the following: "If I had to go out and earn my own living, I doubt if I'd even make a very good cleaning woman. I have no talents, no experience, no training for anything." Although many homemakers in Mrs. Roosevelt's day might have made this type of remark, Mrs. Roosevelt would hardly maintain this view of herself for long. Goodwin (207) describes the evolution of Mrs. Roosevelt's discovery of her talents and strength with the help of her women friends from the League of Women Voters:

> When Eleanor first met [Elizabeth] Read and [Esther] Lape, she was still suffering the effects of having discovered her husband's love affair with Lucy

> Mercer. She sorely lacked confidence. She needed appreciation and she was lonely. She found in Elizabeth and Esther's community of women the strength and encouragement to do things on her own, to explore her own talents, to become a person in her own right.

Evidently, Mrs. Roosevelt succeeded so well in establishing her identity apart from her family that even her mother-in-law rued the transformation. Goodwin (208) comments that "Sara was appalled at the idea of a well-bred women's spending so much time away from home in the public eye. A woman's place was with her husband and her children." Eleanor Roosevelt was no longer the self-doubting woman who fulfilled the duties expected of a well cultivated woman in the home: she had become a self-confident woman who devoted herself tirelessly to work outside the home.

Mrs. Roosevelt enjoyed working outside the home, and she supported women's rights, civil rights, social justice, and other causes. She participated in endless forums and meetings on behalf of the underprivileged sectors of society. She traveled frequently, wrote newspaper columns, and aired radio addresses to the public on subjects such as racism and poverty. Her comments warmed the hearts of many citizens and incurred the wrath of others.

As a public figure, Mrs. Roosevelt tried valiantly to help those who were less fortunate in American society. Yet this was all part of her work life, the forum in which she could easily manifest her compassion and sincerity in return for respect and adoration. Mrs. Roosevelt endured criticism, but she was uplifted and encouraged by the affection and inspiration of her many friends and admirers. Mrs. Roosevelt's work outside the home assured her that her life had value and significance regardless of the state of her family life.

From many perspectives, Mrs. Roosevelt's work life was a refuge from her troubled family life. Mrs. Roosevelt was unhappy as a wife, and she was equally discontent as a mother. According to Goodwin, Mrs. Roosevelt counted eighteen marriages among her five children who survived into adulthood. She felt kinship toward her daughter, Anna, but she did not feel the same toward her sons. Evidently, family life did not provide Mrs. Roosevelt with either a happy or comfortable sanctuary. In contrast to Mrs. Roosevelt's ambivalence toward family life, however, was her unswerving passion for her work outside the home.

It is important to note that as singularly ambitious and intelligent as she was, Mrs. Roosevelt was able to direct the focus of her life from her family to work outside the home because she had tremendous financial security and auxiliary support. She had the assistance of her mother-in-law and abundant hired help to care for her husband and children at all times. Additionally, her homes were replete with many servants, and she had a personal secretary who traveled with her.

Meanwhile, Franklin Delano Roosevelt had a retinue of personal assistants and friends, as well as his mother to attend to his needs. He rarely interfered with his wife's numerous activities outside the home, and he encouraged her to travel so that she could relay to him what she learned from her interactions with the American public. Given these circumstances, Mrs. Roosevelt was in a unique position to establish a new life centered upon her work outside the home instead of the care of her children and her husband.

Ultimately, Mrs. Roosevelt's success in her work life was so extraordinary that she was called "the greatest woman in the world" during the last years of her life. Goodwin emphasizes that Mrs. Roosevelt's success was her own and independent of her husband, the President. Goodwin (209) cites as evidence the five-year contract renewal of Mrs. Roosevelt's news column in 1940, which occurred even before FDR announced plans for renewing his term in office as President. By 1941 she was earning $1,000 per lecture, and her syndicated news column was printed in 135 newspapers throughout the country.

Also, long after her husband's death, Mrs. Roosevelt remained an important political figure. A lifelong New Yorker, Mrs. Roosevelt was well positioned to run for political office, a feat that would have been astonishing for a former First Lady in the mid-twentieth century. Truly, Mrs. Roosevelt was a unique and powerful woman who left the imprint of her achievements on subsequent generations of women.

Mrs. Roosevelt succeeded in her work life at a level that few women then or now could reasonably imagine, but the same cannot be said of her marriage and family life. Understandably, Mrs. Roosevelt's disenchantment with marriage was not wholly unfounded since, as Goodwin notes, it was assumed in that era that one of the primary duties of a wife was to prepare her husband a hot meal for dinner. Male chauvinism prevailed, and some men would not tolerate the notion that their wives could be breadwinners: it was a man's duty to provide for his family while his wife took care of the kids and home.

With such overriding chauvinistic attitudes, it is probable that many women, like Mrs. Roosevelt, were neither satisfied nor content with family life. Thus, when Mrs. Roosevelt lobbied for women to work in munitions factories and plants throughout the World War II era, many women were grateful for her support. In turn, she delighted in meeting women who were thankful to be out of the home and in the workforce. For a pioneering feminist like Eleanor Roosevelt, getting women into the workforce regardless of the work involved was a victory for all women.

A SKEWED VIEW OF FAMILY LIFE

Pioneering feminists like Eleanor Roosevelt nevertheless left behind a legacy that is notable for its markedly skewed view of family life. From Doris Kearns Goodwin's description, the women Mrs. Roosevelt befriended at the League of Women Voters were primarily women without children. They were intellectuals who sought alternative lifestyles that did not include children. Like them, Mrs. Roosevelt placed great value upon work life outside the home. For these intellectual women, the skills learned from working outside the home were more important and valuable than those learned in the home.

In Mrs. Roosevelt's day, many women were relatively uneducated and unskilled. Goodwin (365) quotes Mrs. Roosevelt as saying, "I'm pretty old, 57 you know, to tell girls what to do with their lives, but if I were of a debutante age I would go into a factory—any factory where I could learn a skill and be useful." Her primary hope for women was to encourage them to enter the workforce and develop useful skills. Mrs. Roosevelt would have been pleased to learn that by the turn of the twenty-first century, women comprised nearly half the American workforce. One should question, though, whether even Mrs. Roosevelt would have been satisfied with the gains women have made in their employment outside the home.

Women have gained measurable success in certain aspects of the work world. For example, according to a February 14, 2005, radio broadcast of *To the Point* with Warren Olney on *National Public Radio,* seven Fortune 500 companies have women Chief Executive Officers (CEOs) or presidents whereas there were none a generation ago. The percentage of women who hold at least one-quarter of corporate officer positions at Fortune 500 companies has risen from five percent in 1995 to ten percent (Gettings and Johnson 2005).

Increasingly, women are playing important roles in the field of education: the percentage of women college presidents has doubled from 9.5 percent to 19 percent since 1986 (American Council on Education 2000). There are currently three women presidents of Ivy League colleges whereas there were none prior to 1994. There are also numerous accomplished and well-paid women in various professions, including medicine, law, academia, accounting, journalism, entertainment, and business.

Still, despite the presence of so many hard-working and productive women in the workforce, women's earnings are consistently lower and their positions are less prestigious than that of their male counterparts. In the year 2000, women earned on average about 76 percent of what their male counterparts made (Nightingale and Fix 2004). Also discouraging is the fact that even as more women work longer hours outside the home, many still undertake a far greater responsibility in child-rearing and housekeeping than do their spouses.

Perhaps Mrs. Roosevelt and other feminists should have foreseen the extent to which women would be overwhelmed by undertaking the responsibilities of both family life and work life. However sincere Mrs. Roosevelt's intentions may have been when she encouraged women with young children to join the workforce, she was also disingenuous since she abdicated her child-rearing responsibilities prior to embracing work life. She also had the advantages of wealth that gave her the freedom to choose exactly how she would live. It was precisely because she was financially secure that she could delve into her work life with abandon and relegate the care of her husband and children to other family members and paid helpers.

In contrast, the majority of women today face nearly the opposite situation in that they generally work outside the home in order to accumulate the funds that will enable them and their families to live a more comfortable life. The greater majority of women do not have the financial resources to pursue work life with abandon and hire the high-quality help that Mrs. Roosevelt could so effortlessly afford. Additionally, most women are not focused only on work life outside the home. Consequently, many women work hard both outside and inside the home.

Of course, it is understandable that Mrs. Roosevelt resented the prevailing belief that women of her standing were not to do much beyond marrying and rearing children. This is why she could suggest that young women should learn useful skills, even if they could be used only in factories. The implication is clearly that a woman's talents and skills are manifest primarily and perhaps solely in the arena of work outside the home and not inside the home.

One must conclude that feminists like Eleanor Roosevelt and her friends either did not understand or chose to overlook the fact that the majority of women would wish to have a family life regardless of how much they enjoy working outside the home. The writer Anne Roiphe has commented that feminists failed women by refusing to acknowledge the reality that women would continue to bear children and create families. For many women of childbearing age, work life will not be the single or primary purpose of life. Even so, feminists continue to insist that women will be happy only if they are successful outside the home.

Feminists' emphasis on valuing work life over family life has remained unchallenged for decades. Instead of distinguishing the importance and primacy of family life, feminists have done and still do a great deal to undermine the significance of family life. Feminists may shy away from recognizing the importance of childrearing, but the majority of women will continue to bear children. Whether or not feminists will admit it, the feminist agenda has helped some women greatly, but it has also cost many other women dearly.

One of the unfortunate assumptions that feminists have made is that women would be able to initiate family life at any time whereas women could achieve success in education and work life only in their twenties through their late thirties or early forties. In *Creating a Life: Professional Women and the Quest for Children,* economist Sylvia Ann Hewlett reiterates what anthropologists like Ashley Montagu wrote many decades ago. An unalterable certainty about women's biology is that women are in their reproductive prime in their early twenties. In the meantime, most women have been presuming that they would be fertile throughout most of their pre-menopausal years.

Hewlett notes that there are high rates of childlessness among professional women because many highly educated women prioritize their careers and delay or forgo pregnancy. It is only when they are already in their thirties and forties that some women learn that they are incapable of bearing children. Regardless of advances in fertility research, the experience of enduring repeated, costly, painful, and perhaps unhealthy fertility treatments does not at all guarantee women success with pregnancy and childbearing. Although most infertile women will become reconciled to their infertility, those who had planned to bear children are left to wonder why and how they could not control this aspect of their lives. In response to this realistic portrayal of women's fertility, feminists like the journalist Caryl Rivers accuse Hewlett of presenting an "anti-feminist agenda."

As mentioned earlier, much of today's feminist agenda evolved from ideas that were initiated by feminists like Eleanor Roosevelt and her friends at the League of Women Voters. These women's subjective views of family life have made a lasting impression on succeeding generations of women. Highly educated and financially independent, Mrs. Roosevelt and her friends enjoyed their freedom and ability to achieve so much in life other than mothering and homemaking. In all likelihood, these women anticipated that the majority of women would seek to emulate them and adopt similar goals in life.

BALANCING FAMILY LIFE AND WORK LIFE

It is not at all certain, though, that the greater majority of women are either as ambitious or as driven to succeed only in work life as were Eleanor Roosevelt and her friends. This is not to say that women today are disinterested in either work outside the home or the pursuit of intellectual discourse and stimulation beyond their children and family life. Many women are busy whether they stay home with their children or work outside the home. In fact, it is precisely because women are driven and ambitious that they busily and actively apply their talents to various endeavors (many of which, unfortunately, do not generate income).

Many women use their educational and work experiences to rear their children and volunteer in countless civic and charitable organizations. For example, despite the precipitous decline in the quality of American education, some public schools and many private schools are thriving because women volunteer endless hours by either participating directly in school activities or by overseeing and contributing to substantial fundraising efforts. Many women also play active roles in children's sports leagues as well as community activities. Women join book reading clubs, as well as religious and social gatherings where they can partake in intellectual discourse. In the home, most women manage family finances. In diverse ways, many women are simultaneously involved in child-rearing, work outside and inside the home, and various activities that occupy a great deal of their time outside the home.

Whether or not a woman works outside the home, she may find it difficult to balance family life with all the other responsibilities she may undertake, be it in the workforce or in the realm of volunteer work. The conundrum of balancing family life with work life is one that Eleanor Roosevelt was able to avoid since she did not need to take full responsibility for her family's care. Her successes as a political and social activist occurred after she had fulfilled basic child-rearing responsibilities, and her children were no longer young. Additionally, Mrs. Roosevelt had the financial means to extricate herself from the responsibility of fulfilling her role as a mother and wife.

Work life was of supreme importance for Eleanor Roosevelt since she derived mixed satisfaction from family life. As much as she loved her husband, the limitations of his company exasperated her. When the Roosevelts took a cross-country train trip the year before FDR's death, FDR enjoyed the relaxing excursion while his wife did not. Eleanor's personal assistant entered the following observation in her journal during the journey: "Mrs. R was impatient at the speed and the waste of time" (Goodwin 1995, 528).

According to Goodwin, it is unlikely that Eleanor would have dedicated herself to spending more time with FDR even as he was growing visibly weaker toward the end of his life. Goodwin (528) notes, "Work refused to leave her (Eleanor's) mind…" During the last nine months of FDR's life, the woman who wound up comforting him was his former lover, Lucy Mercer Rutherfurd. Anna Roosevelt, daughter of Eleanor and FDR, arranged surreptitious meetings between FDR and Rutherfurd without informing Mrs. Roosevelt, who was busy with political and social activities unrelated to her family life.

UNDERMINING MATERNAL CARE

Unlike Eleanor Roosevelt, though, most women in the workforce today do not wish to disengage themselves from their identities as mothers and wives. In fact, many women post pictures of their children and spouses all over their work areas because they cherish their family life. During my residency, for example, I had a colleague who used to carry a huge photograph of her toddler under a stack of notes for patients on her clipboard during hospital rounds. The task of balancing family life and work life, while creating value meaningfully in both, is a stressful challenge that many women face every day.

For policy wonks like Eleanor Roosevelt, such a dilemma did not exist because she had little hands-on experience with mothering. From Mrs. Roosevelt's perspective, day care was a suitable alternative to maternal care. After all, day care was merely a form of surrogate maternal care that was probably not too dissimilar from the type of care that she received during her own childhood and dispensed to her own children.

During the World War II era and afterward, Mrs. Roosevelt lobbied strenuously for the establishment of government-sponsored day care centers. She cited legitimate concerns about "a real danger of child neglect" since some women were leaving their young children unsupervised while they went to work. Mrs. Roosevelt encouraged private companies to establish, with government assistance, nursery schools for children of mothers who worked outside the home. The availability of day care would provide children a safe and educational environment while their mothers contributed to the war effort by working at plants and factories.

Goodwin (417) indicates that a model day care institution called the Swan Island Center was built in 1942 by shipbuilders Henry and Edgar Kaiser with funds provided by the U.S. Maritime Commission. Outstanding teachers were recruited, and the center operated six days a week, fifty-two weeks a year. The professional and expert nature of the day care center and its staff were impressive. Goodwin (622) offers a quote from a woman who spoke of the quality of care her children received: "The care and training they received in this child care center is the best possible thing that could have happened to them." This mother's perspective reflected the prevalent understanding that child development experts and educators were more capable of rearing children than were mothers.

After the war ended, Mrs. Roosevelt supported government-sponsored day care for women in the workforce. It made sense to her that women would continue to work outside the home and relegate the care of their children to more expert teachers and staff at professional day care centers. Echoing Mrs. Roosevelt's sentiments, feminists for decades have advocated day care as being the panacea for all families in which mothers work outside the home. They are confident that universal access to day care will enable women of all classes and social backgrounds to ascend career tracks and increase their earnings. This is the assumption feminists make even though there is a dearth of high-quality or even mediocre day care available to the majority of parents, and there is a relative scarcity of high-quality and high-paying jobs for the vast majority of women who are in the workforce.

Singularly focused on keeping women in the workforce, regardless of the age of young children in the home, feminists appear to think that the answer to the problem of child care is to demand government-subsidized day care. Without a doubt, the U.S. government's sponsorship of universal day care in the name of the good of all women and children is farcical. The government is already bloated and inefficient. Besides, the provision of day care does nothing to resolve the single quandary may women face but feminists do not wish to address: How can a mother who loves and wants to be with her young child reconcile her absence from his life because she works outside the home?

TRUE ADVOCACY OF WOMEN'S RIGHTS

As women continue to bear children, many return to work outside the home and leave the care of their young children to others. Although some women may profess no qualms about abandoning their infants and children, many women reluctantly leave the care of their infants to others. The historian Christopher Lasch understood the hardship women faced in pursuing both motherhood and work outside the home.

Lasch was a great champion of women, children, and family life. His book *Haven in a Heartless World: The Family Besieged* encourages women to challenge the status quo and battle for the ascendancy of family life over work life. Lasch (1977, xvii) offers the following insightful comment:

> The problem of women's work and women's equality needs to be examined from a perspective more radical than any that has emerged from the feminist movement. It has to be seen as a special case of the general rule that work takes precedence over family. The most important indictment of the present organization of work is that it forces women to choose between their desire for economic self-sufficiency and the needs of her children. Instead of blaming the family for this state of affairs, we should blame the relentless demands of the job market itself.

Lasch hoped that women would take the initiative to prioritize family life over work life.

Feminists, however, did not seek to ennoble family life over work life. It would have been a huge challenge for feminists to enable women to fulfill the needs of their children and gain equal access to educational and employment opportunities. Instead, feminists ignored child-rearing and emphasized the importance of gaining women educational and employment opportunities. It is evident that feminists did not seek the empowering agenda Christopher Lasch suggested because it was much too radical.

Feminists might have been intrigued by the more radical agenda if they had been at all interested in the well-being of children. Unfortunately, the priority of feminists in the past and today is the same: the focus is on women and their aspiration for sexual equality with men, freedom, and financial independence. Therefore, even though women continue to bear children who need maternal care, child-rearing is a secondary or perhaps tertiary concern of feminists. It is merely a problem that can be solved through the advocacy of universal government-sponsored day care.

Christopher Lasch (1977, xvi-xvii), however, articulates the true dilemma women face but which feminists do not bother to address: "Feminists have not answered the argument that day care provides no substitute for the family. They have not answered the argument that indifference to the needs of the young has become one of the distinguishing characteristics of a society that lives for the moment, defines the consumption of commodities as the highest form of personal satisfaction, and exploits existing resources with criminal disregard of the future." As women continue to bear children, it is becoming more evident that the goals of feminists are limited, and they do not reflect the needs of the many women who wish to care for their own children.

14

WORK LIFE AND ITS CONSEQUENCES

THE DEHUMANIZING CLOCK

The ascendancy of work life over family life leaves many mothers and fathers with little time to spare for their young babies and children. The task of providing hands-on nurturing for even the youngest babies may be allotted to a specific number of minutes each day. The term "quality time" acknowledges both the efforts parents make to be available to their children and the great value of this time, irrespective of its brevity. Time spent with a child, in general, defies the work culture that demands that work outside the home takes precedence over all else, including the care of young babies.

Time is valued so highly that it is measured nearly constantly with the use of watches and clocks. Daily life is organized around the clock, and one hardly considers how it affects one's humanity. Describing how the clock replaced human reliance on the sun and forces of nature, Ashley Montagu and Floyd Matson (1983, xxiii) write that "a peculiar and profound form of dehumanization was taking place, involving the loss of a sense of subjective control or even participation in the conduct of daily life.... Henceforth human life would not move with the tides, but proceed like clockwork."

The historian Daniel J. Boorstin (1985, 36) describes the clock as being the "mother of machines" and notes that the subdivision of the day into hours and minutes occurred in modern times as a result of religious persons in Europe seeking to learn when they should perform their prayers. In many ways the clock so dominates modern daily existence that one can almost sense a religious devotion to the measurement of time.

The dominance of the clock in modern human existence is captured literally in one scene of the 2002 film *About Schmidt*. The actor Jack Nicholson is shown sitting at his desk as he peers anxiously at the wall clock and counts down the seconds to five o'clock. At exactly five p.m., he gathers a box of his belongings, turns off the light switch, exits his office, and closes the door. He is a newly retired insurance actuary whose life is no longer bound by the clock. He soon learns that despite his lifelong dedication to work outside the home, his recent contributions to the workplace have been discarded carelessly into the trash, and he has difficulties communicating with his wife and daughter. His subsequent efforts to spend quality time with his grown daughter are rebuffed and unappreciated.

As parents of even young children consider how to apportion the limited amount of time they have available, the invariable conclusion is that time spent with children is not as productive or remunerative as time spent working outside the home. Thus, many fathers and mothers leave the home in order to earn income. They spend less time with their children and trust that their children will be fine either unattended or in the care of paid caregivers.

In an effort to compensate for their absence, parents may spend quality time with their children. There is, however, nothing inherently valuable about quality time irrespective of parents' good intentions. Parents may wish sincerely to spend meaningful time with their children, but appointed time periods generally lack spontaneity and often feel unnatural, if not forced.

LITTLE TIME FOR MOTHERING

In *The Time Bind: When Work Becomes Home and Home Becomes Work,* sociologist Arlie Russell Hochschild presents three years of research she compiled on employees who work at a Fortune 500 company she named "Amerco." She details the real life stories of employees (whose names she has changed) as they experience daily the reality of how significantly work life overtakes family life. One of the surprises she encounters while doing her research is that few employees take advantage of family-friendly work options that are offered by the company. The majority of employees at this family-friendly company work longer hours than they need to despite the negative impact such work hours has upon family life.

Hochschild describes a successful, middle-aged, hard-working manager at Amerco named Vicky King who works ten hours per day, travels on occasion, and earns more income than does her spouse. Hochschild calls Vicky "an administrative mother" who brings her mothering skills to work and uses her work skills to oversee the care of her two young children at home. Vicky's eight-year-old son is a "good boy" who becomes "more reserved both at school and at home" by the end of Hochschild's research. Meanwhile, the younger four-year-old daughter clings to her mother and often demands more time with her mother. Vicky admits that her office is a refuge from her family and that she goes to her office whenever she wants to escape from them.

Hochschild learns that there are many employees who feel as Vicky does: the refuge in life exists not in the home but at work. Hochschild also cites the case of Linda Avery, a 38-year-old factory shift supervisor who is married and has two children, a 16-year-old daughter from her earlier marriage and a 2-year-old daughter from her current marriage. As soon as she returns home from work, she feels pulled in different directions by the demands of her husband, her unhappy 16-year-old, and the 2-year-old who is still awake when she should be asleep. Hochschild (1997, 38) remarks that Linda "felt she could only get relief from the 'work' of being at home by going to the 'home' of work."

Linda enjoys joking with her colleagues at work and finds home life, in contrast, to be stressful. She also discovers that her husband does more household chores, including caring for their toddler, if she remains at work longer. She discloses the following to Hochschild (38): "So I take a lot of overtime. The more I get out of the house, the better I am. It's a terrible thing to say, but that's the way I feel." Linda thinks she is a better mother and wife by spending less time at home since she can avoid arguing with her daughter and husband.

Meanwhile, Linda uses her motherly skills at work to create a harmonious family-like atmosphere, and Amerco rewards such efforts by recognizing workers who reinforce family-like ties among co-workers. Hochschild (45) perceives that this is not uncommon: "Increasing numbers of people are getting their 'pink slips' at home. Work may become their 'rock.'" Hochschild finds that more women choose to spend time away from their children and husbands, and they prefer to apply maternal intuition and organizational skills toward paid work outside the home rather than toward family life.

Despite Amerco's reputation as being family-friendly, the predominance of work life over family life is pervasive. Even as employees imagine they will foster a productive family life, most wind up enmeshed in a work ethic that demands nearly all their time. Clearly, they do not have enough time to fulfill the demands of both family life and work life. Consequently, many employees find themselves in a time bind that pulls them between two factions of their lives. The result is that family life is often expended inordinately for the sake of leading a successful work life. The fact that this is true for many women employees is significant since the greatest recent growth in employment has occurred among women with young children in the home.

Hochschild accepts de facto the need for women to work outside the home for both financial and personal reasons. Moreover, she does not consider in depth either the mass exodus of women from the home and into the workforce or the young children who are left behind at home or in day care. This line of reasoning is appreciated on two levels by those who advocate the return of women to work outside the home regardless of the age of their children. First, there is the outright assumption that most families today need two parental incomes to support an average middle-class lifestyle. Second, Hochschild invokes the widely accepted belief that women who work outside the home feel better about themselves than do women who choose to stay home with their children.

Citing a few studies from the 1980s, Hochschild (41) makes this striking assessment: "In sum, then, women who work outside the home have better physical and mental health than those who do not." At face value, these studies probably reflect the reality of living in a consumer-oriented society: most individuals will probably feel better about themselves if they are paid for their work. It is understandable that women who earn an income from working outside the home may feel more fulfilled than women who work in the home without pay.

If one examines a bit more in depth the nature of such fulfillment, however, one may perceive that the self-assessment of "better physical and mental health" may be illusory. Will the same women feel similarly content when their children turn out less ideally than they expected? What if these children could have benefited from receiving more maternal care, but their parents were simply too busy working to even notice their children's needs? Ultimately, it may be disingenuous to cite repeatedly the importance of earned income in bolstering women's self-esteem. This increased self-esteem, in the long run, has little to do with the actual well-being of young children or their mothers.

Although Hochschild accepts the reality that women work outside the home and may feel better about themselves, she is also aware of the link between poor child development and the long hours many parents work outside the home. Hochschild (10) even quotes the economist Sylvia Ann Hewlett who has written that the long parental workday has led to alarming trends in child development. These negative outcomes include underperformance in school, suicide, need for psychiatric help, severe eating disorders, bearing children out of wedlock, taking drugs, and becoming victims of violent crime.

Hewlett offers somber observations, but Hochschild does not criticize parents for failing to offer their children sufficient parental care. At best, she acknowledges the fact that many mothers and fathers feel guilty about not spending enough time with their children. Evidently, the fact that parents feel guilty should be sufficient proof of parental concern and dedication.

Hochschild argues that parents do not have the time to address all of their children's needs. In any case, the children's physical needs are being met since they are cared for by babysitters, day care centers, or other family members. If, on the other hand, one looks at the children's behavior as it is presented by Hochschild, it is clear that they are in need of greater parental attention. She notes that the children ask for more attention but that the parents are simply too preoccupied with work to respond to their children's requests.

Hochschild recognizes the children's suffering, but she does not address it since the compelling subject at hand is the angst that the children's parents experience. Children may demand parental time and attention, but they will probably not receive it. Even as parents argue that they are doing their best for their children in spite of the time bind, there is little assurance that parents are actually doing a good job of parenting.

INEFFECTIVE PARENTS

Overall, *The Time Bind* presents parents as being good workers but ineffective parents. This makes sense since practice makes perfect. When parents spend a great deal of time at work perfecting the art of working, they may wind up spending so little time with their children that it is almost impossible to perfect the art of parenting. While many parents may feel guilty for not parenting well because of severe time limitations, others have no such qualms.

The Escallas, for instance, are a blue-collar couple who work full-time and overtime at Amerco. Deb Escalla offers Hochschild (185) this remark about her children: "Maybe it's just my kids, but they're a wild bunch. Gina whines an awful lot. Hunter is a very stubborn girl. I think I'd rather be working. When I took a few months off, I just felt like I had to get away. If work's what you have to do to get away, so be it. Plus, I'm getting paid for it." Mario Escalla sympathizes with his wife and admits that he cannot tolerate staying home with their three children since they cause trouble constantly. When the couple head to work at Amerco, they deliver their three children (who are 1 ½ years to 5 years old) to the care of various family members.

Both Deb and Mario perceive work outside the home to be more relaxing than dealing with and relating to their children at home. Deb also believes that if she chooses to stay home with her children, then her husband would help her even less at home, and she would lose her financial independence. Even though Deb and her husband received the benefits of maternal care, Deb confides to Hochschild (185), "I thought about staying home with the kids, but they drove me nuts."

Hochschild (191) offers an astute analysis of the Escallas' situation when she comments that a conflict had arisen between Mario and Deb: "A gender war for time was underway in which the real losers were their children. Implicit in this war was the devaluation of the work of raising children." Deb and Mario view the work to be done in the home, including the care of their children, as an obligation the other must bear.

Although the conflict appears to be sequestered within the Escalla family unit, all three children will eventually enter the educational system and society at large. If it should happen that the Escalla children mature into dysfunctional students and adults, it is unlikely that their parents would reflect too harshly upon themselves. After all, they would be assured of the fact that they worked long hours outside the home for the sake of their family.

THE ADVENT OF "MAKE-WORK"

The dilemma presented by the Escallas' "gender war for time" is a consequence of a view of work, "make-work," that has been promulgated since the era of the New Deal. The objective of make-work is to keep people working so that they can sustain consumerism, which in turn keeps people employed and encourages increased production (Lasch 1997, 10). As long as people consume goods and services, the drive for increased production and employment continues. This is a self-perpetuating cycle that requires more consumers and more workers even though most of the consumption and work are blatantly redundant and unnecessary.

One or two generations ago, the economy functioned fine with one-income families. The current economy, however, encourages two-income families simply because of the sheer volume of make-work and consumption. The main consequence of dual-income families, in which both parents are immersed in make-work and constant consumption of goods and services, is that many parents do not have the time to care for their children. What has happened in the current economy is that many parents work to legitimize the existence of make-work even though they may need to sacrifice the care of their young children.

Undoubtedly, parents may be misled into trusting that this work is of greater importance than the work of caring for children since make-work is both income-generating and seemingly productive. Immersed in and committed to performing make-work, many parents assume that they are doing the best they can for their children. Much of this has to do, of course, with the increased income that supports both a better lifestyle and provides children with access to better education and more entertainment.

As mentioned earlier, many fathers in the past went to work outside the home, earned family income, were often absent from the home, and left the task of child-rearing to their wives. Today, many mothers may offer similar justification for leaving the care of their young children to others. In a society that revolves around make-work, it may be true that two incomes are needed to enhance a family's lifestyle and parents' ability to fund their child's educational opportunities. At some point, nevertheless, serious consideration must be given toward understanding the negative impact that make-work and the absence of parental care may have upon children's development.

TROUBLED CHILDREN

A huge market for substitute caregiving has arisen as a result of the increasing number of babies and children who are no longer cared for by their parents or relatives. The U.S. Department of Labor offers the following optimistic job outlook for child care workers:

> High replacement needs should create good job opportunities for childcare workers. Many childcare workers must be replaced each year as they leave the occupation to take other jobs, to meet family responsibilities, or for other reasons. Qualified persons who are interested in this work should have little trouble finding and keeping a job. Opportunities for nannies should be especially good, as many workers prefer not to work in other people's homes (U.S. Dept. of Labor 2005).

The U.S. government expects a strong and continued demand for low-paid child care workers.

It is unclear how many babies and children will be the recipients of care that is disbursed in a high turnover job market by low-paid employees with variable educational backgrounds. Granted, there are talented and affectionate caregivers who may be poorly educated and low-paid. Then again, there are also individuals who should never be employed in child care. The cost of caring for babies and children in this unpredictable manner is becoming evident in unexpected ways.

For instance, the incidence of childhood psychiatric and behavioral problems has risen dramatically. Fifteen years ago, children were placed on anti-depressants as a last resort for chronic bed-wetting. In contrast, anti-depressants are now prescribed to hundreds of thousands of young children and adolescents who are suffering from depression. According to the National Institute of Mental Health (NIMH), up to 11 percent of young children and adolescents suffer from depression, and 50 percent of those children have another psychiatric disorder (Boykin and Harper 2004). In the meantime, attention deficit and hyperactivity disorders continue to afflict an enormous number of youngsters, increasingly at younger ages.

The November 17, 2002, issue of the *New York Times Magazine* features an article about a controversial federal government study of Ritalin use in three-to five-year-old preschoolers. Parents of one child who is in the study claim they can tell from his behavior whether he is taking Ritalin or a dummy pill. The child's parents are convinced of their child's need for medical intervention. Understandably, many parents and physicians place great emphasis upon treating mental illness in children with medications. After all, it is difficult to elucidate the causes of mental illness since there are many genetic and social variables involved in determining the outcome of youngsters' development.

MISUNDERSTANDING HEREDITY

Ashley Montagu (1959) clarifies in his textbook *Human Heredity* that every individual is born with two types of heredity: genetic heredity and social heredity. Genetic heredity is often mistakenly accepted to be an individual's sole heredity as if genes alone determine every aspect of an individual's life. Also, genes are frequently thought to be fixed traits that are unalterable in their expression. Such an understanding of genes, however, is limited since it overlooks the enormous impact a child's social heredity has upon the expression of genetic potential. Without the proper environmental stimulus, genetic potential may remain unexpressed.

For instance, I know a professional violinist whose life had taken a turn toward the cinema and photographic arts. Her sons did not demonstrate a musical proclivity until they began receiving formal music lessons, whereupon they displayed immediately their musical talent. Until my friend created the environment in which her sons could manifest their genetic potential to play string instruments, their ability to create music remained dormant and untapped.

It is the social heredity that provides the individual with the environment in which he will grow and develop. This environment includes not only the physical womb in which the embryo matures into a fetus but also his parents, immediate and extended family members, home, community, country, and the planet Earth. The importance of social heredity cannot be underestimated because everything in a child's environment helps to determine how his genetic potential will be expressed.

Recent scientific research corroborates the importance of the environment even on a microscopic level. This can be seen, for instance, during the in vitro fertilization protocol that is commonly used to treat infertility. A harvested egg and some sperm are placed into a culture medium so that they can fertilize to produce an embryo. Very small and seemingly insignificant alterations in the chemical environment of a developing embryo have been found to cause genes to behave unexpectedly.

According to Rosie Mestel in the January 24, 2003, issue of the *Los Angeles Times*, researchers Richard Schultz and Marisa Bartolomei at the University of Pennsylvania found that small changes in the culture medium, like the amount of salt or amino acids used, can cause the genes in the embryo to turn on when they should be off and vice versa. This research demonstrates how significantly small changes in the physical environment affect even the gene expression of an embryo. Additionally, it has been noted that children who are born via in vitro fertilization have a higher incidence of Beckwith-Wiedemann syndrome, an overgrowth disorder that is grossly visible and easily detectable.

Mestel notes that scientists are now concerned about "subtler errors involving complex traits and genes for which there are no tests." Research on the microscopic level demonstrates that there are inconspicuous and perhaps unknowable influences that the environment can wield upon genes. Thus, greater attention needs to be paid to the social heredity, on both the microscopic and macroscopic levels, in which young babies and children grow and develop.

THE ALTERED SOCIAL HEREDITY OF CHILDREN

As mentioned earlier, it is rarely acknowledged that the social heredity of young children in the U.S. has changed dramatically over the course of the past century.

Not only has breastfeeding been eliminated from many children's social heredity but so has hands-on maternal care. For the duration of human existence, a child's social heredity more or less included the presence or availability of his mother since breastfeeding was integral to human survival.

As a result of the changes wrought by industrialization and the advent of relatively safe artificial milk substitutes for infants, however, both breastfeeding and maternal care have become somewhat obsolete. In other words, the widespread use of infant formula has altered indelibly the social heredity of nearly every individual born in the U.S. over the past century. Young babies and children over the past century have been the recipients of care that differs markedly from the care that countless forebears received in early childhood.

Although babies and children appear to be surviving, it does not necessarily mean that they are either happy or fulfilled. In fact, babies cry a great deal in protest, but most parents ignore babies' crying. Then, when children are old enough to vocalize their complaints, parents may interpret such behavior as manifestations of willful or spoiled temperaments. Understandably, many parents may see little need to address legitimate concerns about the well-being of their young children when it is evident that they are surviving in the absence of breastfeeding and maternal care.

In many ways, a baby's survival is no longer a major source of concern for increasing numbers of parents. In fact, some parents are so confident of their baby's well-being that they place their unborn baby's name on waiting lists to attend prestigious pre-schools. Other parents may determine early on which elite private college their child will attend. What is taken for granted is not only the survival of babies and children but also their ability to manifest the wonderful genetic potential they inherit from their parents.

Indeed, some parents are so confident of their own achievements and the genes they have passed on that they feel assured that their children will surely demonstrate similar success in life. This is due, in large part, to the fact that many parents are more affluent than were their own parents. Parents today can afford to bestow upon their children material advantages that they could not have conceived of receiving during their own childhood.

Overall, children today receive significantly more toys, educational support, clothing, accessories, and access to entertainment than did most children of previous generations. One friend remarked a few years ago that he was concerned that his wife went overboard when she bought their seven-year-old son approximately thirty Christmas presents. Parents today understand well the importance of providing their young children with security and comfort. The same cannot be said of parents' appreciation of maternal care and its role in healthy child development. This is a shame since maternal care often assured most children's healthy survival and well-being.

The majority of women throughout history were able to provide their children with maternal care. What was possible for most women in the past was the concurrent ability to work productively within or near the home and rear their children. Most women were accessible to their breastfeeding children even as they worked outside of the home or nearby the home for most of human history. Sadly, work now often takes many women far away from home and their young children, and it is usually incompatible with the provision of hands-on maternal care.

Such incompatibility between work and child-rearing is, however, being challenged. Pam Belluck reports in the December 4, 2000, issue of the *New York Times* that some companies are willing to permit their employees to bring infants directly to work with them. Kathleen Sebelius, the Kansas insurance commissioner who authorized this policy for 160 employees three years earlier, tells Belluck: "It just allows a parent to be a caregiver. It doesn't involve all the production of having a day care center, with the cost or licensing or liability. Parents don't have to make choices about, 'Am I a parent or am I a worker?' And people are nicer to each other if there's a baby around." Belluck cites the success of this policy for fathers and mothers in various settings, including a bank in San Jose, a law firm in Chicago, a personnel agency in Fort Lauderdale, Florida, and a university in Richmond, Virgina.

In the May 3, 2005, issue of the *New York Times*, Melinda Ligos reports that some women are bringing their babies to complex work settings. For instance, Alana K. Bassin is a Minneapolis-based partner of a law firm who brought her breastfeeding seven-month-old baby to a trial in Texas for two weeks. Bassin informs Ligos, "When I tell senior male partners at other firms that I do this, they're shocked. They can't believe I'd bring a baby across the country with me, especially to a trial, which they liken to going to war." Bassin's determination to breastfeed and care for her daughter as she works in a demanding profession is encouraging.

Employers and employees alike can help to set a precedent for other women who wish to participate actively in the work world while bringing nursing children along. Unfortunately, most employers (irrespective of gender) are uninterested in promoting flexible work schedules for mothers. Hence, the maternal care that was once available to the majority of children is now something that fewer families are willing or able to afford.

Obsessed with the scarcity of time, many parents tend to think about the needs of their young children, but they do not act to secure the satisfaction of such needs. Hochschild mentions in *The Time Bind* that all the parents she interviewed think about their children and family life, but most do not take the action to enhance the quality of family life. Merely thinking about doing things for a child, however, is not equivalent to actually making the effort and taking the time to do something with a child. It takes great effort and determination to provide maternal care in a culture that demeans the work of mothering.

Parents may convince themselves that their children's genetic endowment and an abundance of goods and procured services will assure their children's healthy development. This is a delusion since human beings are complex and intricate biological specimens. Irrespective of modern cultural trends that ignore mothering, children need their mothers. The absence of maternal care in many children's social heredity is an egregious but correctable deficiency.

15

STAY-AT-HOME MOTHERING

HAPPINESS AND MOTHERHOOD

A baby's birth is a momentous occasion that generally arouses an indescribable sense of love, joy, and commitment from the baby's parents and family. The happiness that accompanies the birth of a healthy baby is emotional and all-encompassing. At times, however, the birth of a healthy baby may not register sustained awe and appreciation of life.

The birth of a child has become in some ways an event to mark with specific rituals. Prior to the birth, pregnant women are often feted with a baby shower and a plethora of gifts; after the birth, mothers are presented with flowers; and yearly afterward, the day is celebrated with gift-giving and perhaps parties. Even though the birth itself is a huge and significant event, many women no longer have enough time to establish a definitive relationship with their babies. This is particularly true for women who return to work outside the home soon after taking brief maternity leaves.

Although the norm today may be the early separation of babies from their mothers, this was hardly the custom for most of human existence. For example, writer Anita Diamant offers a fictional account of childbirth during Biblical times in her novel *The Red Tent*. When one of the women is about to give birth, all the other women in the family (including other wives of the baby's father since polygamy was a cultural norm) set aside their personal differences and jealousies. They work together to support the childbearing mother by massaging her, applying herbal ointments on her body, feeding her, and responding to all her needs while she experiences the challenges of giving birth.

Once the baby is born, the mother is pampered and celebrated as a bearer of life. The women indulge the breastfeeding mother with carefully prepared and nourishing foods and bolster the mother-infant dyad. They support her emotionally by caring for her physically and permitting her to rest. They offer their services to the mother so that she may be available to her newborn child. Although this is a fictional narrative, many women throughout human history probably gave birth not alone but in a supportive setting similar to the one Diamant suggests.

Women today can find support for childbirth through natural childbirth education and the assistance of doulas. For the past few decades, natural childbirth classes and informative books have enabled husbands to take an active role in the childbearing process. The advent of doulas, women who coach pregnant women during labor and encourage the mother-infant dyad after childbirth, is relatively new in the U.S. A doula's knowledgeable assistance may alleviate a pregnant woman's fear of childbirth and help to initiate the breastfeeding relationship. Few women, however, are either aware of doulas or can afford such helpful services during childbirth.

For the most part, women today wind up giving birth with their spouses, friends, or alone in inhospitable hospital settings. New parents may also be distanced geographically or emotionally from other family members as a consequence of job relocations, frequent moves, or purposeful estrangement. Thus, many new parents may not receive much auxiliary support as they experience the life-altering experience of welcoming a newborn into their lives.

There may even be times when a baby's birth is either taken for granted or perhaps resented. This is undoubtedly perplexing and discouraging for the approximately 15 percent of American couples who find that it may be difficult or impossible to become pregnant and bear babies (Barad 2004). Impaired fertility is prevalent enough that there is a very strong demand for artificial reproductive intervention.

Many thousands of women who wish to bear children have undergone or are undergoing fertility treatment. The costly and perhaps harmful intervention of fertility protocol nevertheless cannot at all guarantee successful pregnancy or childbearing. The reality of childbearing in modern society is that while infertile couples hope desperately for the birth of a baby through the use of medical technology, there are other couples who may not truly appreciate the birth of a baby.

The modern era is unique since more parents have the time and opportunity to contemplate the meaning of life: they can determine what will bring them some measure of satisfaction and happiness in life. Regardless of how simple or difficult childbearing may be, some women may find the task of child-rearing to be unfulfilling. Therefore, they may wish to pursue whatever they think will bring them greater happiness while they offer their children less than attentive care or relegate their children's care to others.

This line of thinking and approach to child-rearing contrasts starkly to the way of life most women led in the long history of human existence. In the past, women had little or no time to think of anything beyond work and survival, which included child-rearing. Happiness was not necessarily an objective in life but simply a byproduct of hard work and great suffering. In marked comparison, instead of perceiving happiness to be an earned privilege, many now consider happiness to be an inalienable, and often unearned, right.

The historian Christopher Lasch remarks that when Betty Friedan wrote *The Feminine Mystique*, she was writing specifically about the disenfranchised housewives who lived in the suburbs and were preoccupied with the contemplation of their misery. Although Friedan's focus was on women and their lack of fulfillment, Lasch opines that the true ordeal women faced was the physical and cultural isolation of living in the suburbs. Lasch (1997, 105) describes life in the suburbs as follows:

> Domestic servants, extended family members, friends and neighbors acting as an informal support system—all were excluded from the middle-class suburban household, with the result that housewives found themselves in sole possession, free at last to arrange things exactly as they pleased. It did not take long for this freedom to pall. By the early sixties (if not before), the "holy refuge" of the suburban family came to be experienced as a "comfortable concentration camp," in Betty Friedan's memorable phase.

Women living in the suburbs learned that their responsibilities in the home could occupy only a limited amount of their time, energy, and intelligence. Consequently, the frustration and despair they experienced were attributed not to the loss of the extended family and community ties but to the fact that they were at home rearing children. Henceforth, it would be assumed that a woman who chooses to stay home with her children would be no different from the frustrated and unhappy 1950s suburban housewife.

DEPRESSION IN THE ABSENCE OF BREASTFEEDING

The elimination of breastfeeding from child-rearing practices has arguably had a more pervasive and harmful influence on the well-being of women than the impact of living in the suburbs. By the 1950s the role of breastfeeding had been nearly obliterated from child-rearing practices. Whereas breastfeeding had provided mothers an incomparably unique role in their babies' lives throughout the long history of human existence, the widespread use of infant formula obviated the womanly art of breastfeeding. Without the need to breastfeed, it became clear that many of the roles fulfilled by mothers could be performed by anyone else, including relatives or hired help.

The overriding view of mothering today is that the work of a mother can be, and perhaps should be, performed by anyone other than a mother. It is widely assumed now that mothers do not possess responsibilities that are unique to them, particularly during a child's infancy. Of course, mothers are told that they are special, but they are not appreciated for doing the work of hands-on mothering.

After all, it seems that poorly paid helpers can perform child-rearing tasks as well as mothers: they can display affection, change diapers, feed infant formula, speak and play with babies, hold them, take them for a stroll in the carriage, and put them to sleep. Hired helpers can also cook meals, clean house, and do laundry. With the significant exceptions of a woman's ability to breastfeed, offer personalized love, and perhaps be a role model, it may be argued that there is nothing exceptional about a mother's role in her infant's life.

As reiterated frequently throughout this book, however, the absence of breastfeeding in child-rearing practices can no longer be overlooked. Breastfeeding is a unique activity that is specific to women. Ignoring this most basic function of women's biology engenders unnecessary risks to the health and well-being of far too many babies and their mothers.

In recent years, growing attention has been paid to the incidence of "baby blues" or mild forms of postpartum depression. It is estimated that 40 percent of the four million U.S. births that occur annually are complicated by some form of postpartum mood disorder (Leopold and Zoschnick 2005). Unfortunately, few researchers or parents pay much attention to either the medical intervention that often disrupts mother-infant bonding or the biological anomaly of women choosing not to breastfeed.

As infertile women undergo fertility treatments, more women are subjecting their bodies to artificially induced hormonal changes that may not be benign. Suffice it to say that women's behavior is most certainly affected by hormonal changes. For instance, when women are afflicted with Premenstrual Syndrome (PMS), they may suffer from a variety of symptoms, including mood swings and physical discomfort. This phenomenon with its associated hormonal changes may recur regularly with every menstrual cycle. One may surmise that fertility treatments might also affect women's behavior significantly as they attempt to conceive, succeed in conceiving, and then undergo the experiences of pregnancy, childbirth, and motherhood.

Additionally, many women may choose not to breastfeed without comprehending how highly beneficial and long-lasting the hormonal changes that accompany breastfeeding may be for both infants and mothers. The hormones that accompany the physiological process of breastfeeding have far-reaching and profound consequences upon the well-being of both infants and their mothers. Research continues to elucidate the benefits of hormones that are associated with childbearing and breastfeeding.

For instance, oxytocin is a significant hormone that induces labor in childbirth, returns the uterus back to its pre-pregnancy size, and permits the milk to be ejected from the breast during breastfeeding. Benedict Carey, in an article entitled "Hormone Dose May Increase People's Trust in Strangers" in the June 2, 2005, issue of the *New York Times* notes that Swiss scientists have determined that the administration of oxytocin "can consistently alter something as sensitive as trust." Carey writes, "The new finding could help researchers not only understand the biological system underlying social judgments but also perhaps correct it when it goes awry, as in conditions like social phobia or autism, scientists say." Although some scientists are wary of placing too much confidence in oxtyocin's ability to create trust, what is evident is that biological changes are associated with the creation of trust and other human behaviors.

Other research demonstrates that oxytocin appears to influence human beings' ability to bond with one another later in life. Oxytocin has been shown to play a major role in attachment: it is released during sexual climax, childbirth, and breastfeeding. Science writer Steven Johnson (2003) writes that some scientists think that the release of oxytocin "during important pair-bonding events helps cement the image of a partner or a newborn in the mind's eye. The biological capacity for love helps the brain prepare humans for offspring who are born young and helpless and require tending to have the slightest hope of survival." The tending or attention given to offspring is manifest as social bonds between parent and child, the parents, and other caregivers in the family. These social bonds are reinforced on the biological level by the presence of oxytocin, which provides pleasure, reward, and satisfaction.

The recognition of a biological basis for the mother-infant bond is important since it may explain, in part, why some mothers may feel detached from their babies despite loving them. In the absence of a healthy pregnancy, childbirth experience, and breastfeeding, it is possible that a woman might not experience the biological basis for the mother-infant bond that is integral to a healthy mothering experience. Without such a biological foundation, it may be that much more difficult for a woman to enjoy her experience as a mother, no matter how much she may consciously wish to love her baby.

As with everything in life, a mother's mood is not static but dynamic and affected strongly by many internal and external variables, including the hormonal influences of pregnancy, childbearing, and breastfeeding. Although women may find that they need fertility drugs or face obstetric intervention with childbirth, they may be able to mitigate disruptive consequences of such interference with mother-infant bonding by breastfeeding. Although breastfeeding is considered to be an optional mode of infant feeding, it is actually a vital tool to help women to fulfill their maternal role in child-rearing. Modern culture, regrettably, does not have a healthy regard for the biology of breastfeeding.

In a culture that does not embrace breastfeeding, it is possible that maternal happiness may be elusive. As mothers continue to detach themselves physically from their young babies, a skewed view of womanly happiness develops: a woman's happiness is perceived to be something that is distinct and apart from maternal happiness. A woman's happiness, however, is determined not just by conscious will or desire, but very crucially by biology and the natural function of breastfeeding. In the absence of breastfeeding, women may find neither happiness nor fulfillment in child-rearing, in homemaking, or in life for that matter.

THE WORK OF MOTHERING

The work of mothering and housekeeping can be challenging and burdensome. Increasingly, women (and some men) who are disenchanted with the work of parenting and housekeeping have begun maintaining a blog, which is a journal that is kept online and made accessible to the general public. Danny Hochman offers the following observation in an article entitled "Mommy (and Me)" in the January 30, 2005, issue of the *New York Times*: "Parents have never waited longer nor thought more consciously about having children, yet time and again the bloggers voice surprise and sometimes resentment about the unglamorous reality of bringing up baby."

The work of child-rearing and housekeeping may be tedious and unexciting enough for some parents to forget a basic reality of life: every significant human activity requires effort and work that may be for the most part repetitious, seemingly uneventful or meaningless, and perhaps unenjoyable. Undoubtedly, much of the anguish associated with parenting is simply because it is unpaid work, and there is so much of it to do. It is impossible to offer an accurate assessment of how much a woman's work is worth in the home.

An informal study performed by a Web site called Salary.com, however, determined the following: "Stay-at-home mothers wear many hats. They're the family CEO, the day care provider, accountant, chauffeur, counselor, chef, nurse, laundress, entertainer, personal stylist, and educator. Based on a 100-hour work week, Salary.com has estimated that a fair wage for the typical stay-at-home mom would be $131,471 for executing all of her daily tasks" (O'Brien 2005).

Lena Bottos, compensation market analyst for Salary.com observes, however, that the compensation still does not adequately measure a mother's work in the home. She says, "When you take into account that it represents a 100-hour workweek, and doesn't even begin to factor in that they are on call 24 hours a day, it's not so large. Plus, stay-at-home moms get no benefits in terms of pension or 401(k)" (O'Brien 2005).

Jennifer Steinhauer reports in the May 8, 2005, issue of the *New York Times* that Edelman Financial Services measured the value of a busy mother's work by adding the salaries of 17 different workers and came up with a figure of $707,126. This seems to be an outlandish figure, but it is an accurate valuation of a mother's work. The hands-on rearing of a healthy child is far more valuable than the work, for instance, of a Chief Executive Officer (CEO) whose corporation manufactures and distributes guns, tobacco, alcohol, or junk food. Obviously, these are subjective judgments, but the fact remains that a mother's work is misunderstood and unremunerated.

As a whole, the true value of stay-at-home mothering cannot be assessed accurately since the value of a woman's availability, organizational skills, efficiency, responsiveness, and interest are immeasurable. It is impossible to find a single person to replace the work and efforts of a capable and hard-working woman in the home. Consequently, the solution for some families may be to replace a woman's work in the home through piecemeal efforts.

HOMEMAKING

Several years ago in the *New Yorker* magazine, Margaret Talbot wrote about hired helpers who do some of the work that mothers would ordinarily do inside and outside of the home. Talbot describes hired helpers who do far more than clean house and help with child care. Cleaning house and child-rearing are tasks that have long been delegated to low-paid housekeepers and nannies. The persons Talbot describes are well-educated and well-paid individuals who presumably possess good taste and a talent for shopping, decorating, and planning.

These paid helpers undertake tasks that an upper-middle class mother might fulfill on an ordinary day, such as shopping for personal or decorative items for use at home or as gifts. They also have good organizational skills, so they can oversee lifestyle choices like arranging and decorating personal belongings in clients' homes. Moreover, they can handle details associated with arranging dinner parties and social gatherings for their clients. These are activities that women normally do in the home as part of maintaining family life and home life, but professionals can now offer their expertise and services for a fee.

Talbot describes other services that were not needed a generation ago. For instance, there are drivers who shuttle young children from school to after-school activities like karate or gym class and then home since most children participate in activities that are not located near their homes. Dependence upon these hired helpers is costly but apparently worthwhile for those who can afford them.

As more women have become preoccupied with income generation outside the home, fewer women have the time to do the work of maintaining their homes. Notwithstanding the ubiquity of efficient washers, dryers, vacuum cleaners, and dishwashers, it takes effort and work to keep a home clean and tidy. Although some women may enjoy doing housework because it provides exercise and results in a cleaner home, other women are frank about their distaste for housework.

Cooking is a domestic responsibility that is a bit different from house cleaning although kitchen clean-up is integral to cooking. While some women may abhor the thought of cooking, others do not have the time to enjoy cooking. As a result, even though more homes today feature pretty and well-equipped kitchens, including state-of-the-art appliances, many kitchens remain curiously unused. According to an article in the *New Yorker* magazine a few years ago, Viking, the manufacturer of upscale kitchen appliances, plans to offer cooking lessons in order to encourage its clients to use the costly appliances they purchase. Apparently, homeowners pay thousands of dollars to outfit their kitchens with stunning appliances that are rarely, if ever, used.

The fact that many families are not cooking at home is reflected in the booming sales of frozen meals and freshly prepared deli foods that are offered by grocery stores and supermarkets. Even high-end restaurants are now offering fully prepared meals that can be delivered curbside for patrons to pick up and eat at home. With little time to spare, fewer women are engaged in creating and encouraging family meals at home.

The traditional family dinner is no longer part of the average family's schedule. "The family that eats together stays together" is a quaint adage since few families have the time to eat meals together. When families do have an opportunity to eat together in the home, the meals may often consist of pre-cooked or frozen food that has been heated for dinner.

Although the work of cooking may not be appreciated, cooking at home may be instrumental in preventing serious cases of food poisoning. Surveys done by the restaurant industry claim that more cases of food poisoning occur in the home than in restaurants or store-prepared foods. This may be true if home cooks do not practice safe cooking measures such as frequent hand washing; proper handling of meat by washing hands, chopping board, food preparation surfaces, and utensils in warm water and soap afterward; and making sure that meat and vegetables are fresh and safe to consume.

With proper education, home cooks can feed their families safely and more nutritiously than can restaurants or grocery delis. Discouragingly, millions of people watch popular television cooking shows that may actually increase ignorance of proper food handling techniques. Frank C. Rizzo notes in the July 8, 2004, issue of the *Atlanta Journal-Constitution* that one study of American cooking shows found that an average of seven food-handling mistakes are made on a 30-minutes show. This is unfortunate since television cooking shows may perpetuate poor food handling practices among home cooks.

As it stands, 76 million cases of food poisoning occur annually in the U.S. (Wrong Diagnosis 2003). The majority of cases are not serious, but the elderly, individuals with compromised immune systems, and young children are the most susceptible to bad outcomes. In an era when dining out has become a way of life for numerous families, it is inevitable that the risk of food poisoning increases.

In Los Angeles, city inspectors make diligent efforts to grade restaurants for cleanliness and the way in which workers handle food. The *Los Angeles Times* reported recently, however, that inspectors must pour bleach over tainted meat in order to prevent restaurant workers from fetching the spoiled meat from the dumpster and cooking with it. Although the restaurant industry will claim that such behavior among food workers is aberrant, it occurs with enough frequency that food inspectors in Los Angeles need to take definitive measures to prevent such actions from sickening restaurant patrons. In contrast, it is highly doubtful that a conscientious home cook would use tainted meat or food to cook for family members or friends.

Additionally, an important reason to avoid dining out is that the nutritional value of the food that is offered to young children is questionable. Purveyors of fast food are notorious for luring young children into their establishments by advertising widely on television the desirability of free toys that accompany the purchase of children's meals. Parents are aware of the junk food these fast food restaurants offer. In comparison, parents often do not consider the low quality of food that is offered to young children at sit-down restaurants, including those that are expensive and rated highly. Most children's menus offer the least healthy or the most inexpensive food that any dining establishment can offer its patrons.

Ostensibly, restaurants try to serve foods that children would enjoy eating, like French fries, cheeseburgers, hot dogs, pizza, pasta (with butter and cheese), macaroni and cheese, chicken fingers, soda, juice, and ice cream. All these foods, however, are either highly processed or high-fat foods that contain inordinately large amounts of salt or sugar. The sole green vegetable offered to young children is the parsley garnish that will undoubtedly remain uneaten.

On the other hand, parents who cook at home can oversee their children's diets and regulate the types of foods that are eaten. Parents can also shop for specific foods and eliminate undesirable food items. Although fathers may not have much time, they can participate actively in this particular aspect of child care by shopping for food and cooking once the baby is six months old and eating solid food.

Undoubtedly, many men and women are busy, and they may contend that they have more important things to do than spend time on banal aspects of domesticity. Consequently, some families may tolerate a more slovenly lifestyle while others may pay helpers to do domestic work. Although women in the past might have been content with or at least reconciled to the value of rearing children and keeping house, the same cannot be said of women today.

THE VALUE OF MOTHERING

In the modern era, maternal care and mother-infant bonding are expendable even though the constant interaction between a loving mother and her baby leads to the baby's first healthy socializing experience. Many parents take it for granted that their babies will develop into healthy and caring children as long as they are given adequate physical care. Unbeknownst to most parents, this is a relatively new and unproven assumption. In fact, it was shown long ago that the positive social interaction between a baby and her loving caregiver is of immense importance to a baby's survival.

According to the historian Salimbene, thirteenth century German Emperor Frederick II tried to determine which language babies would speak in the absence of receiving any verbal stimulation from their caregivers (Montagu 1986, 101–102). The emperor ordered foster mothers and nurses to suckle and care for the babies but not to "prattle with them." He wondered which language the babies would speak spontaneously, whether it would be Hebrew, Greek, Latin, Arabic, or their parents' language. Sadly, the experiment was an abysmal failure. Salimbene writes, "But he laboured in vain because all the children died. For they could not live without the petting and joyful faces and loving words of their foster mothers." Ashley Montagu relays this historical account in his book *Touching* to affirm the importance of the affection and touching that encourage the healthy development of babies.

Parents today may not appreciate the significance of this historical experiment since it appears that babies survive despite the absence of breastfeeding and maternal care. With the widespread availability of sanitized water and commercial infant formula, survival for most infants is assured. Besides, most parents will not purposefully subject their young children to the care of cruel and unloving substitute caregivers. Instead, they will try to provide surrogate care that is modeled closely upon loving and competent maternal care. In addition, when parents are available, they will surely give their children loving attention and care. Thus, the reason that most babies do survive is that their parents care a great deal about their well-being.

The questions that need to be asked, however, are the following: If a baby ideally needs loving maternal care, which may be given in the form of high quality surrogate care, why is hands-on maternal care expendable? Why should a mother not provide her baby or young child with the loving care that will best suit his growth and development? These questions remain unaddressed although some will declare emphatically that women have better things to do than stay home to mother young children.

Current child-rearing practices indicate that there is no grand vision of ensuring greater women's rights that would include the right and responsibility of a woman to mother her child and maintain her home. Instead, there is an overwhelming urgency to get as many women as possible to succeed and gain fame in the work world. Such a goal may definitely be reasonable and possible for childless women, but it is profoundly more challenging, if not impossible, for women with young children.

Presently, what is believed to be achievable by all women is dictated by a minority of women who have chosen either not to have children or to have children and relegate their children's care to others. This means that women who wish to stay home with their children may be unwittingly and uncomfortably placed in a defensive position. They may need to explain why they are not following the feminist agenda.

What has happened is that the majority of women now face relentless pressure to conform to standards in family life and home life that have been set by a minority of women who claim to represent all women. Under the guise of liberating women from the banality of domesticity, feminists have long discouraged women from becoming attached to their babies. For far too long, feminists have overemphasized the need for all women, including mothers of babies and young children, to remain in the workforce.

The seriousness with which feminists have neglected mother-infant bonding is exemplified in the failure of the National Organization for Women (NOW) to support legislation that would have required employers to grant parental leaves in the mid-1990s. NOW, the stalwart feminist organization, reasoned that women would probably take the leaves, perpetuate the division of labor that force women to assume greater responsibility for child care, and inhibit women's professional career advancement (Lasch 1997, 118).

Feminists have long battled for women's rights, but many of the gains have been made at the expense of both children and their mothers. For instance, by denying women's need to take a more primary role in rearing children, feminists undermine a basic biological and singular need for mothers and babies to breastfeed. In truth, it is utterly incomprehensible that the mother-infant dyad lost its unique status as a profoundly special relationship in an effort to advocate women's rights. After all, what could possibly be as special as motherly love for and devotion to the baby a woman carries in and bears from her womb?

Feminists may argue against mother-infant bonding because they think that women need to be relieved of the burden of staying home. In a way, one can understand the superficial aspects of this line of reasoning. There are times when it may be unclear as to what a baby needs, and this can be frustrating for women who approach their lives in a business-like fashion. A baby's growth and development may appear to be remarkably slow and uneventful, especially in the first year of life. Additionally, and perhaps frustratingly, the physical care of an infant may frequently be demanding, untidy, and imprecise.

The fact remains, nevertheless, that women continue to bear babies. The majority of women are obviously not bearing babies simply because they believe it is an unnecessary burden. Many women wish to become mothers. Thus, if feminists are to represent all women, then they should proclaim and defend the importance of a woman's responsibility, right, and need to care for her own child as a mother.

16

THE ART OF MOTHERING

MATERNAL SACRIFICES

It has been politically incorrect for many years to suggest that women need to make sacrifices in order to rear their children. This is comprehensible since no one wishes to be taken for granted. It is hard, however, to argue that a baby or young child takes his mother for granted when he seeks fulfillment of his most basic needs. Fundamentally, it is unfortunate that human beings evolved to begin life in such a profoundly needy and helpless state.

Human beings do not possess the instinct to care rightly for their progeny, and in the absence of such an instinct, parents must learn how to care for their own children. They must also decide what kind of sacrifices they will need to make on their children's behalf. In order to offer babies ideal care, which should include the benefits of breastfeeding and maternal care, it is usually women who wind up making most of the sacrifices. Women may find this to be disturbing and, thus, most discussions of maternal sacrifices do not revolve around the positive and beneficial effects such sacrifices have upon the well-being of children, their mothers, and their families. Instead, what is emphasized is the burdensome nature of maternal sacrifices and its negative impact upon women's self-identity.

Psychologist Carin Rubenstein wrote a book called *The Sacrificial Mother: Escaping the Trap of Self-Denial,* and she begins the book by describing her dilemma with pickles. In the author's home, everyone loves to eat pickles; when it comes down to the last pickle in the jar, she carefully slices it so that the other family members each get an equal share. Rubenstein declines to partake in eating the last pickle and evidently no one ever offers her a piece. Then she notices one day that even though she makes sure that all the members of her family are dressed well, she wears tattered sweats, and her hair is untidy.

Rubenstein performs surveys and discovers that many women become sacrificial mothers who deny themselves a great deal. The primary point of her research is that women wind up making unappreciated sacrifices too often at the expense of their self-esteem. It may be true that mothers may become sacrificial and neglect their own needs, but it is similarly valid nevertheless that the same women can develop common sense in order to comprehend their own needs and limitations. Rubenstein, for instance, resolves the pickle dilemma and learns how to balance maternal devotion with her own needs and issues of self-esteem.

Since women continue to bear children who need to be reared, it is imperative that women comprehend the basis for healthy and meaningful sacrificial behavior. True concern for the well-being of babies and children arises from altruism, which is a profoundly important state of life that represents the human capacity to do for others or to make sacrifices without necessarily thinking of oneself or one's own needs. Without altruism, the survival of most creatures, including human beings, would be imperiled.

Petr Kropotkin offered his insight as a field observer who observed cooperation and mutual aid in nature more frequently than he saw competition. His various essays, which were compiled in *Mutual Aid* in the late 1800s, include the following important passage:

> And man is appealed to be guided in his acts, not merely by love, which is always personal, or at the best tribal, but by the perception of his oneness with each human being. In the practice of mutual aid, which we can retrace to the earliest beginnings of evolution, we thus find the positive and undoubted origin of our ethical conceptions; and we can affirm that in the ethical progress of man, mutual support—has had the leading part. In its wide extension, even at the present time, we also see the best guarantee of a still loftier evolution of our race (1976, 300).

The hope for humankind is to envision, as Kropotkin does, the greater development and nurturing of compassion, goodness, and consideration.

Such humanity is readily displayed by loving and caring mothers daily throughout the world. Unfortunately, it has become commonplace to denigrate the natural practice of mothering young children. Modern child-rearing practices tend to ignore the significance of maternal care, and they do not espouse Kropotkin's vision of a "still loftier evolution" of human beings.

MOTHERING, GUILT, AND RESENTMENT

The art of mothering is being lost without considering how short-sighted it is to assume that a woman's success in life is determined by how much income, fame, and status she accumulates outside the home during her twenties, thirties, and forties. There is no reason why a woman cannot enjoy such successes later in life, most notably after she has completed responsibilities associated with child-rearing. This is particularly true since the average American woman lives into her mid-seventies.

Throughout human history, motherhood and its numerous and attendant responsibilities were integral to most women's existences. What is markedly different today is that motherhood or childbearing is still a vital part of a woman's life, but the work of mothering is not. For many women, the work of mothering is something that needs to be done after the fulfillment of occupational, financial, social, or personal obligations that are unrelated to the care of their children.

Since the vast majority of women experience work as something that is incompatible with child-rearing, work frequently takes them out of the home and far away from their children. As many women embark on the path of pursuing both child-rearing and work outside the home, many realize that it is impossible for them to do everything excellently both within and outside the home. This may be discouraging for the many women who try their best to do everything well. On the other hand, a minority of women may be able to do many things well simultaneously.

Allison Pearson, for instance, is an award-winning journalist, bestselling author of the novel *I Don't Know How She Does It*, mother of two young children, and the wife of film critic and writer, Anthony Lane. Pearson is the prototypical hard-working, high-achieving, and successful supermom who has managed to succeed in journalism, writing fiction, and fostering her family life. She also accepts without question the need for women with young children to work outside the home.

Apparently, Pearson decided long ago against providing her children with hands-on maternal care. In a November 5, 2002, interview that was published in the *Los Angeles Times*, Pearson reveals the following: "'All I knew was that I didn't want my mother's life,' says Pearson, who says her mother was woefully overqualified for housewifery. 'There are two kinds of mothers: resentful and guilty. I'd rather be guilty.'"

This is a facile view of motherhood that emphasizes overwhelmingly its negative aspects. The reality of life is that regardless of how guilty or resentful mothers may be, they may also be fulfilled, happy, dedicated, unresentful, and altruistic. This is, in any case, irrelevant since it is simpler for Pearson to define motherhood as being an experience that engenders either guilt or resentment.

Pearson opines that an intelligent and talented woman is too qualified to be only a mother and homemaker. In a sense, she may be correct since many women have talents that can surely be directed toward diverse activities other than mothering. At the same time, one must ponder the unique responsibility that a mother has for her child. Additionally, one would think that talented and intelligent women have even more to offer their children. Pearson nevertheless trusts that such women should exert their energy elsewhere and not toward child-rearing.

The irony is that Pearson received maternal care and undoubtedly benefited immensely from it. Even so, she probably sees no correlation between her success in life (as a loving mother and wife, award-winning journalist, celebrated novelist, and more) and the care she received as a child from a mother who, however resentful she might have been, still stayed home to care for her children.

In a May 2003 interview with Bookreporter.com and in answer to the question of how it is possible for one family to have "two high-powered parents," Pearson (2003) replies, "What you need is really good childcare." Pearson was probably fortunate to have found and hired high-quality substitute care for her children. Although Pearson may perhaps feel guilty at times, one assumes that she does not feel resentful.

Women like Pearson are unusual since they succeed at a level that few women can even contemplate, let alone aspire to achieve. Such success, however, cannot be attributed simply to talent, intelligence, and ambition since both luck and timing are critically important as well. Although a few women are graced with an unusual combination of the varying factors that determine immense success, the vast majority are not. In other words, supermoms like Pearson are uncommonly lucky, and they should not be held up as role models for the majority of women. Pearson may claim that she prefers to feel guilty, but what she actually advocates is maternal indifference toward young babies and children.

UNMINDFUL OF MATERNAL DEPRIVATION

In order for Pearson to dismiss the importance of maternal care, she must assume at least two things: First, she must think that the growth and development of her young children will not be impaired by her absence, and second, her children will know that she loves them. Pearson (2003), in fact, tells her Bookreporter.com interviewer that she dedicated her novel to her six-year old daughter because it was her way of saying, "This is how your mother's generation had to live and never think I didn't love you."

Unfortunately, Pearson's comment is disingenuous because she does not have to live this way. Rather, she deliberately chooses to live this way since she prefers to feel guilty instead of providing her children with hands-on maternal care. Like many other parents who disregard the importance of maternal care, Pearson is gambling that maternal deprivation will not affect adversely the growth and development of her young children.

The relevant question that needs to be addressed is the following: Who exactly is observing and determining what the healthy growth and development criteria are for young babies and children? Undoubtedly, parents, family members, and pediatricians will all agree that the majority of children are growing and developing well and normally. It will astonish parents nevertheless to learn that highly educated and objective professionals can be wrong when it comes to assessing behavioral development.

For instance, in her book *Love at Goon Park: Harry Harlow and the Science of Affection*, science writer Deborah Blum (2002, 214) describes the work of behavioral psychologist Harry Harlow. In one experiment, Harlow subjected baby monkeys to a surrogate mother that repeatedly rejected them. The babies returned constantly to the rejecting mother, and Harlow was convinced that he had failed to elicit psychotic behavior from the baby monkeys.

Around that time, the psychiatrist John Bowlby visited Harlow's laboratory. Bowlby had theorized the importance of attachment between child and mother after observing over a long career the devastating signs of maternal deprivation among British children who were separated early in life from their mothers; children who were hospitalized and separated from their mothers; and disturbed adults who as children had been separated for safety reasons from their parents during World War II (Garelli 2004).

Bowlby observed Harlow's maternally deprived and rejected monkeys sucking and cuddling themselves, as well as rocking their bodies back and forth. Bowlby recognized immediately the signs of maternal deprivation in Harlow's laboratory monkeys. He told Harlow, "You've got some crazy animals" (Blum 2002, 214).

Astoundingly, even though Harlow was a well-trained and highly experienced behavioral researcher, he missed seeing blatant signs of maternal deprivation in his experimental monkeys. Who can deny that pediatricians and other child-rearing experts, who are as experienced and professional as was Harlow, may similarly be unable to perceive the devastating effects of maternal deprivation on young children who have not received consistent and loving maternal care?

The effects of maternal deprivation on young babies and children are very evident, but it has become politically incorrect to state the obvious: there is something amiss with the behavior of many young children today. This is the case since current norms of child-rearing already include significant amounts of maternal deprivation. Simply stated, behavior that is assessed to be normal today would have been considered to have been abnormal just a generation ago. Increasingly, the standards of acceptable and normal behavior are becoming more complex and muddled.

Consider the vociferous and angry response to day care researcher Jay Belsky's recommendation that young children spend less time in non-maternal care. He found that children who spent more than 30 hours in non-maternal care per week were more likely to display behavioral problems in Kindergarten. Peggy Orenstein offers this remarkable comment in her article entitled "Bringing Down Baby" in the April 29, 2001, issue of the *Los Angeles Times*: "A closer look reveals the statistics to be less alarming. Only 17% of children in day care showed 'explosive,' 'disobedient' or 'aggressive' tendencies, which means the other 83% did not. What's more, the differences that do exist are well within the realm of normal—day care hardly breeds school shooters. And since 9% of children who stay home with mom are also seen by their teachers as aggressive by kindergarten, the real differential is only 8%."

Orenstein assesses that it is acceptable that nearly one in six children in day care demonstrates uncooperative and perhaps harmful behavior. Although she makes light of an 8 percent differential between aggressive children in day care versus aggressive children who received maternal care, she overlooks the fact that day care produced nearly twice as many children with noticeable behavioral problems. Orenstein's analysis of children's behavior is both absurd and frightening since she chooses to ignore the startling news that 17 percent of children in day care behave abnormally. Instead, she glorifies the fact that 83 percent of children in day care behave normally.

Orenstein, an inveterate pro-day care advocate demonstrates misplaced optimism, as does day care researcher Alison Clarke-Stewart. Orenstein writes, "'These are little differences' in behavior, insists Alison Clarke-Stewart of UC Irvine. 'If the results showed that 50% of children in child care were more aggressive, I would agree that's something we need to be concerned about. But 17% is what the test predicts as normal in the general population.'" Evidently, Clarke-Stewart will not be concerned until half of children reared in day care demonstrate overt behavioral problems.

Clarke-Stewart offers an unhelpful and simplistic analysis of the data, which Orenstein notes in her article: "As Clarke-Stewart points out, many factors could account for the disparity. For instance, she says, mothers who stay home may be less aggressive than those who work and so tend to raise more docile kids." This suggestion is silly since it assumes that women at home are less aggressive than women who work outside the home even though nearly all women have been trained in the same male-oriented educational system and work arenas. Clarke-Stewart may not be aware of how aggressive some stay-at-home mothers can be. For instance, I once cringed during a gym class for toddlers when a stay-at-home mother suddenly got up and called out loudly for her robust twin daughters to put greater effort into running after a much smaller, frightened boy during a routine play exercise.

The issue that should be addressed is the presence of behavioral problems in even 9 percent of children who have been reared in the home by their mothers. This is not a subject that is raised since day care advocates need to downplay the troubling evidence that day care creates even more troubled children. Evidently, pundits like Orenstein and Clarke-Stewart deem this rise in children's poor behavior to be normal. What they are effectively suggesting is that parents need not be concerned about the widespread occurrence of behavioral problems among young children, at least not until half of children display such problems.

The faulty analysis of data on day care and children's behavior does not help the many parents who undoubtedly love their children. Parents are reassured by day care advocates that it is fine to choose to send their young babies and children to day care instead of providing them with maternal care. Consequently, parents will do their best for their children and entertain hopeful and positive thoughts about their children's well-being.

Unfortunately, a mother's cerebral and sincere love for her baby may not be able to compensate for her frequent absence from her baby's life. After all, a young baby or young child cannot differentiate maternal absence from maternal rejection. Simply stated, it is highly doubtful that a baby will know how much a mother loves him if she is simply not there for him.

If, as Allison Pearson suggests, it is better for women to feel guilty rather than to make sacrifices, many women are feeling guilty already. Yet what is the good of feeling guilty? It is well known that by making some sacrifices, a mother can do her best to prevent her children from experiencing maternal deprivation. What more does one need to know?

THE PRACTICE OF MOTHERING

In defiance of common sense, it must now be proven unequivocally through objective scientific studies that a baby needs his mother. When such studies are performed and duly demonstrate the importance of maternal love and availability in a child's life, accusations of bias are made. The validity of these studies, however, cannot be ignored regardless of how antithetical they may be to current feminist ideology.

The psychologist Harry Harlow and his colleagues performed numerous studies on animal behavior in the 1950s, and they were able to demonstrate the importance of maternal love, maternal availability, and tactile stimulation to healthy infant development (Montagu 1986, 40). In one of many studies he performed, Harlow placed baby monkeys in a cage that contained two surrogate mothers that were made of wire mesh. One was covered in cloth and was incapable of ejecting milk while the other was not covered in cloth and was capable of ejecting milk. Harlow's experimental baby monkeys clung constantly to the cloth surrogate who could not provide milk; when they were hungry, they reached over to the wire mesh surrogate to drink milk.

At the time these studies were made, the prevailing understanding of maternal availability was related primarily to the literal act of feeding a baby. Freud had postulated that infants were attached to their mothers because it was the mothers who generally fed them. What Harlow's numerous studies clarified was the significance of the touch and the love that accompany the mother-infant relationship during feeding. Harlow's studies showed that a baby monkey needs much more from his mother than mere oral nourishment. In numerous studies performed at Harlow's psychology laboratories, it was evident that the gold standard of monkey rearing was to permit a baby monkey to hang on to his mother and nurse freely.

Although an abundance of scientific evidence supported the recognition of a mother's unique role in her child's life, much of it was dismissed by the women's movement. Feminists argued that the research and theories that advocated the importance of maternal care were a ruse in the name of science to get women to stay home. Both John Bowlby and Harry Harlow were vilified by the women's movement.

Deborah Blum (2002, 235) describes the unusual predicament Bowlby and Harlow faced: "It wasn't just being attacked that was so upsetting. Both Bowlby and Harlow had endured years of that from their own colleagues. They could shrug off a few insults. It was the irony of it, the injustice. Why should they be criticized for saying that mothers mattered, that the female of the species was loved, needed, and extraordinarily influential? Why should they be harassed for saying that children mattered?" Blum describes the paradox perfectly: women's advocates disparaged two men who recognized and appreciated the uniqueness of a woman's role in child-rearing.

One has to surmise that women who were angered by Bowlby and Harlow either did not have children or they were uninterested in the well-being of children. Why else would women argue against recognizing the specific and special role a woman fulfills as a mother? It is ultimately both curious and discouraging that feminists were not interested in exalting the right of women to behave like women.

Throughout human history, there have always been a minority of women who were disillusioned with child-rearing and its attendant obligations. What is astonishing, though, is how widespread this cynicism toward hands-on mothering has become even as women have continued to bear children. At this time, a minority of mothers breastfeed and care directly for their babies, and one may conclude sadly that many women are suppressing their maternal intuition. Moreover, many women appear not to be aware of the plethora of evidence that demonstrates the significance of mother-infant bonding for both babies and mothers.

If one repudiates mother-infant bonding while advocating any care for babies other than a mother's care, then one should consider how the denial of mother-infant bonding affects mothers. Ashley Montagu (1986, 42) writes eloquently, "When a baby is born a mother is also born." This does not mean merely that a woman becomes a mother when a baby emerges from her womb. Rather, it means that a woman's identity as a mother is born, and it is ready to grow and develop. This perception of motherhood identifies clearly how little any woman knows or understands about being a mother until she actually becomes a mother and does the work of mothering.

Ultimately, it does not matter how much knowledge a woman acquires about child-rearing since knowledge without wisdom is meaningless. The Buddhist philosopher Daisaku Ikeda (2000, 1:15) writes, "Though knowledge can be transmitted from one person to another, wisdom cannot. The only way to develop wisdom is to acquire it through personal experience." The wisdom of mothering develops and accrues through the practice and experience of mothering.

THE SUPPRESSION OF MOTHERLY INTUITION

Most mammalian mothers are inseparable from their newborns because they are driven by instinct to protect their babies. This was illustrated by Harry Harlow in one of his earlier psychological experiments. He built a device that separated hungry mother rats from their babies, and he divided them with a mesh barrier that contained small holes that were large enough for the babies to pass through but too small for the mothers to squeeze through (Blum 2002, 23).

During the experiment, the baby rats were confused, so they wandered aimlessly in circles. Meanwhile, the hungry mother rats ignored food that was offered as a distraction, and instead focused single-mindedly and desperately on trying to get to their babies. As soon as the mesh was lifted, the mother rats raced to gather and protect their babies. This experiment demonstrated clearly the mother rats' instinctive drive to protect their babies.

While human mothers do not possess instincts, human mothers indubitably feel protective of their children. Such a maternal drive was illustrated in the Biblical tale of King Solomon's wisdom in resolving a dispute between two women who both claimed to be the mother of the same baby. He proposed cutting the baby in half, sagaciously understanding that the real mother would never agree to such a plan. In general, it is the anomalous mother who expresses indifference to her baby. Like the frenzied mother rats that were willing to do anything to protect their babies, most human mothers unquestionably feel a similarly strong kinship toward their offspring.

In the absence of instinct, women possess the intuition to protect their babies and children. Women tend more often than not, however, to restrain themselves. For example, when my son was in the Neonatal Intensive Care Unit (NICU), I wanted to scold a sick nurse who came to work one day even though she was sneezing and coughing. After being cared for by this nurse, my young two-week old prematurely born son became ill with a viral infection, and he required yet more medical intervention. His delicate skin was poked and prodded repeatedly for blood tests and an I.V. site. His physician stopped his oral feedings of breast milk and let him subsist on a less than nourishing I.V. solution of sugar and amino acids for a few days. I could do nothing for my son even though I was as frenzied as were the mother rats in Harlow's experiment.

Harlow's experimental rats were more candid and fearless than I was in their willingness to demonstrate their love for their baby rats. In contrast to the expressive mother rats, women are civil, composed, and willing to go along with the flow of cultural norms. It would have been disrespectful of me, after all, to accuse the sick nurse of making my son ill. I was supposed to be respectful by suppressing my maternal drives and viewing my child's care with objectivity. Therefore, I was dutifully cooperative and tried to act as detached as possible.

When women approach motherhood with aloofness, however, healthy urges to care for their babies may be deliberately subdued. Child-rearing may even become an instructional and cerebral activity rather than an intuitive and emotional interaction with one's child. In the long run, women would be better off if they trusted their own intuition, the internal feeling of right and wrong that one derives from experience. Like the hungry mother rats that ignored the available food and chose to protect their babies instead, it is probable that more human mothers would act similarly protective and make more sacrifices for their children if they did not stop to think too much.

17

THE CONTEMPORARY MOTHER

IMPERFECT MOTHERING

As mentioned frequently before, what is right and good for babies often conflicts with what parents think is best for themselves and their lifestyle. Parents in the distant past might not have had the time to think too much about what they needed to do to ensure their babies' survival and well-being. In contrast, in the modern era, a great deal of thought is expended by many parents who question exactly how much they need to do for their babies and children.

Babies and young children, then, are at the mercy of parents who might or might not be able or willing to provide them with optimal and nurturing care. The current state of parenting is, to say the least, precarious. It is almost as if even imperfect mothering cannot be given a chance because it is simply not worth the bother. It is a terrible shame that the art of mothering might be lost because it is deemed to be either too difficult or not worthwhile.

Regrettably, there are indications that more parents are willing to abdicate their responsibilities when it comes to child-rearing. In an age when divorce is common, it is almost absurd to suggest that parents should consider the well-being of their children first. The well-being of children may almost become an afterthought for some parents. Thus, in support of parental custody rights, children under the age of five years may fly alone across the U.S. (albeit under the supervision of flight attendants) to see one of their divorced parents. Clearly, parental rights often outweigh the needs of children.

Marriage or motherhood for some parents may simply be a phase of life that ends arbitrarily. In the 2002 comedy film *Orange County*, the father of the protagonist regrets divorcing his first wife. He assesses her to be a better mother than his much younger second wife, and he decides to return to his first wife. The second wife drives up in her sports car, approves of their impending divorce, hands over their toddler son, and rushes off to a nightclub: motherhood is over for the younger woman. In the interim, the husband and his toddler are welcomed happily by his first wife. This is a fictional account of modern marriage, and it is no doubt a satire, but it is hardly a reassuring view of family life.

THE NEGLECTED MOTHER

Literature often reflects accurately the condition of human beings for a given time period. Many contemporary novels depict the modern day suffering of women and correlate the emptiness in these women's lives to their unhappiness with family life. At the root of many of these fictional characters' discontented state is resentment as well as either an inability or unwillingness to appreciate the value of family life.

In *Ladder of Years*, novelist Anne Tyler writes about a middle-aged woman who leaves her physician husband and three children, a high-school aged son and two young adults. The woman, Delia Grinstead, abandons her family one day by moving to another town and starting life anew on her own. Without taking notice of the confusion and hurt she inflicts upon the family she leaves behind, she assumes her new identity as a woman beholden to no one.

While Delia is alone and unfettered by the needs of others, she develops an entirely new lifestyle that is centered upon fulfilling her own needs. She finds a job and manages to survive well on her own. Delia reads, eats sparingly but nutritiously, exercises regularly, sleeps plentifully and soundly at night, and lives frugally. She learns how to enjoy her life by satisfying only her own needs.

One can sympathize with Delia because she marries soon after finishing high school and becomes a wife and homemaker. She assumes, like many women did in the past and some still do, that marriage and child-rearing will bring her happiness. Then, suddenly at the age of forty, Delia decides that her life is so profoundly unsatisfying that she deserts her husband and three children.

In a sense, the family has drained Delia of her vitality, and she has become a stunted human being whose existence is marked by emptiness and a lack of joy. Meanwhile, strangers in the new town find her to be endearing. They seek her friendship, and the reader perceives that Delia has much more charm than her family appreciates. Ultimately, Delia manages to succeed in fostering healthy self-esteem because she is ostensibly courageous enough to detach herself from her undeserving family.

THE BORED AND DESPAIRING MOTHER

Another contemporary fictional character who faces an identity crisis similar to that of Delia Grinstead is Laura Brown in Michael Cunningham's novel *The Hours*. Like Delia, the way in which Laura can establish her self-identity is to seek personal satisfaction away from her family. Laura is in such despair about the meaning of her life as a pregnant 1950s Los Angeles housewife that she contemplates suicide.

Laura Brown is a fictional character who is supposed to emblemize the quandary faced by many women who lived in the suburbs in the 1950s: she is an intelligent woman whose talents and ambitions are constrained by marriage and motherhood. Whereas Delia had aspirations of happiness from marriage and child-rearing, Laura feels only ambivalence toward family life.

Mere interaction with her young three-year-old son engenders stressful, existential angst. For instance, Laura is overwhelmed by a multitude of emotions when her son helps to bake a birthday cake for his father. He spills some flour, and she senses his extraordinary sensitivity as well as his need for reassuring love. Laura would like to leave and "be free, blameless, and unaccountable," but instead she assures her son that it is fine that he spills flour (Cunningham 1998, 78).

When Laura sees that her son is relieved, she feels encouraged and empowered enough to resolve the following: "She will not lose hope. She will not mourn her lost possibilities, her unexplored talents (what if she had no talents, after all?). She will remain devoted to her son, her husband, her home and duties, all her gifts. She will want this second child" (79). Laura Brown determines to be a good mother and wife, but she cannot persuade herself for long that she must fulfill these responsibilities.

The unhappiness the fictional Laura Brown experiences is supposed to represent the nearly universal misery of countless 1950s suburban housewives. These women's desolation and the oft told story of their despair strongly influence the modern perception of what mothering can and should be today. Feminists, for instance, balk at the suggestion that women today might wish to apply their talents and skills toward child-rearing and homemaking. It is as if feminists' vision of motherhood is irrevocably enmeshed with the intractable image of an unfulfilled 1950s suburban housewife. This is the case despite the fact that this particular period of child-rearing was incredibly short in comparison to the long history of human existence.

By the 1950s breastfeeding had been nearly eradicated from American child-rearing practices. If women breastfed in that era, they usually did it in secret and without the approval of their babies' pediatricians. At that time, and still today, it was generally understood that by eliminating breastfeeding from mothering responsibilities, women were seemingly freer both physically and emotionally from their children.

This is why, in effect, Laura Brown could look at her toddler with such detachment and ponder intellectually her son's fragile nature. In reality, this had little to do with her obvious intelligence. More accurately, the cerebral and removed way in which Laura interacts with her son reflects the longstanding influence of child-rearing experts: for decades mothers had been encouraged to suppress maternal intuition and empathy. Sadly, women today are left with the legacy of unhappy and disengaged mothers of earlier generations and a distorted view of the maternal role in child-rearing.

MOTHERS FROM THE RECENT PAST

In light of such unhappy fictional portrayals of mothers, women today cannot help but hope that they do not become similarly wretched. This is certainly true of contemporary women whose own childhoods were marred by their mothers' imperfections and misery. If one leafs through the recent memoirs of currently prominent women, one can perceive how they recall their mothers with a mixture of compassion, admiration, disappointment, detachment, and frustration.

Ruth Reichl, a well-known food writer and currently the Editor-in-Chief of *Gourmet* magazine, describes her mother in her memoir *Tender at the Bone: Growing up at the Table*. Readers are introduced to Reichl's mother with a combination of humor and pathos. An inveterate and unremorseful server of spoiled food who causes countless cases of food poisoning, Reichl's mother is intelligent, energetic, and bizarre. She is eventually diagnosed to have a manic-depressive disorder. Reichl (1998, 34) recalls the following: "My mother had lots of energy and education and not a whole lot to do. 'If only my parents had let me be a doctor,' she often wailed as she paced the apartment like a caged tiger."

Throughout this book and the second installment of Reichl's memoirs, *Comfort Me with Apples: More Adventures at the Table*, the image of Reichl's mother is that of a domineering and insufferable woman who insists always that she is right. She is driven to fulfill her own needs constantly while she ignores the needs of her husband and children. Thus, she is able to go abroad for one month with her husband while leaving her sensitive six-year-old daughter in the care of the child's grandmother, who could not tolerate the company of children. She predictably sends the child away to the care of a non-relative; meanwhile, Reichl's mother enjoys her vacation abroad.

Another woman who was subject to comparable or worse motherly neglect is the writer Anne Roiphe. She portrays her mother in withering terms in *Fruitful: A Real Mother in the Modern World* (1996, 5): "She had no work in life other than the beauty parlor, the shopping lists, the decorating of the house.... She had servants for the real work of the home. She cried herself to sleep most nights. She yearned and did not know what she yearned for."

Roiphe (5–6) also describes poignantly how she used to wait to catch a glimpse of her mother: "I have written it many times. I can't seem to stop. I come back to it in novels, in stories, in articles. I started writing my first novel with the picture of a child waiting outside a closed door. The child was me. I would lie on the carpet outside her room, my face pressed to the crack under the door through which I could see the blankets on her bed rising and falling. I didn't play. I didn't move. I waited, my back pressed to the wall so nothing could grab me. She was there but I couldn't reach her." Like Ruth Reichl, Anne Roiphe describes her mother as being a woman who had such vast and unfulfilled needs that she had little interest in being a mother.

Yet another prominent woman who writes about her mother is Jill Ker Conway, the historian and first woman president of Smith College. In her memoir *The Road from Coorain*, Conway recounts how her family thrives briefly in the harsh deserts of Australia. Unfortunately, their sheep ranch is subjected to an unrelenting and prolonged drought. After years of facing seemingly insurmountable difficulties and a succession of challenges from a harsh and uninviting environment, Conway's father commits suicide. The family is devastated by this unexpected event, but Conway's intelligent and resourceful mother is able to persevere.

Conway's mother manages to care for her children and the family's finances. She is savvy and astute enough to hold on to her ranch even though she and Conway move back to the city. Over the ensuing years, regrettably, Conway's mother cannot focus her energy and talents on a worthwhile occupation.

Conway's mother devolves into a woman who takes her deepest frustration out upon her own children. Conway (1989, 231) describes how her mother ousts Conway's brother and his family from her house after she accuses her daughter-in-law of damaging a piece of furniture: "My mother was now an angry and vindictive woman, her rages out of all proportion to any real or imagined slight. She was most destructive toward her own children, especially where she had the power to damage their relationship to others."

A nurse by training, Conway's mother had been a most capable and efficient woman on the ranch. She changes significantly, though, after her husband's suicide: she becomes a woman who cannot perceive anyone's needs other than her own. So willfully contemptuous is her mother that Conway feels compelled to leave her native land and travel halfway across the world to find fulfillment in life.

The mothers described in these memoirs were miserable, and it must have been difficult and perhaps agonizing for these intelligent women to recount such unhappy childhoods in their memoirs. Also, it is evident that their mothers, possibly with the exception of Conway's mother when she was younger, did not necessarily enjoy being mothers. Motherhood or the nurturing aspect of being a mother appears not to have been an integral aspect of these women's identities.

It should be noted that Conway's mother breastfed her children and was a hands-on mother who cared intimately for her children. She took the well-being of her children seriously and proudly, and by all standards was an excellent mother. Sadly, her husband's suicide would forever influence how she would mature later in life as both a woman and a mother. Regardless of how nurturing she might have been early on, Conway's mother changes, and she becomes, from her daughter's perspective, almost diabolical.

Breastfeeding and stay-at-home mothering are only two aspects of being a mother. Neither is a panacea that guarantees indefinitely the well-being of a mother, child, or family. Such an assurance cannot be made since relationships are built upon continual efforts to build and sustain loving interactions. As long as such efforts are made, breastfeeding and stay-at-home mothering can surely provide an indispensably important foundation for prolonged family stability.

Regrettably for Jill Ker Conway, the challenges her family faced were overwhelming enough to cause great sadness and discord in family life. Yet despite having experienced such adversity, Conway succeeds at a level that is remarkable for a girl who was home educated through elementary school. Conway's mother, irrespective of the sadness and anger that consumed much of her own life, did have a measurably positive influence on her daughter's life.

A WOMAN'S SELF-IDENTITY

As evidenced by these examples of fictional and real-life women, a lack of self-identity is a profound source of suffering for women (and men, no doubt). The perennial challenge for women is to be able to develop and maintain a strong sense of self-identity. Fundamentally, women who possess a strong awareness of their self-identity have conviction and a sense of purpose in life.

Regrettably, recent generations of women have experienced identity crises, and it has been assumed that their unhappiness was related to the limitations of their roles as wives and mothers. These women, however, were troubled by significant social changes that affected their ability to mother. Most momentous of these changes was the development of what the historian Christopher Lasch calls the "proletarization of parenthood," which was discussed earlier in Chapter 12. Social forces that included social workers, psychiatrists, educators, penologists, physicians, and psychologists invaded the private domain of family life in the name of knowing what was best for the average American family. As long as women were indebted to such external authorities for child-rearing advice and for solutions to their domestic problems, many women must have wondered what role they actually needed to play in their children's lives.

For example, Anne Roiphe's mother could offer the impersonal support that financial security provides whereas her daughter was merely hoping to receive the intimacy of love and affection. Or in the cases of Ruth Reichl and Jill Ker Conway, their mothers wound up reversing roles with their daughters. Their mothers sought succor and support from their daughters without reciprocating either genuine appreciation or respect. These writers' mothers were simply too self-absorbed to acknowledge the needs and accomplishments of their daughters.

The mothers of these writers were profoundly self-centered and incredibly helpless in so many ways. It is as if they had no idea how to expend their energies and talents productively. For these women to exert themselves in some meaningful way toward the responsibility of mothering appears not to have been a real consideration. At best, all these women could do well was to complain about having nothing worthwhile to do.

It would be disingenuous, however, to suppose that so many women were miserable only because they were not permitted to work outside the home. In truth, a constellation of factors contributed to women's lack of fulfillment over the past century. Women might have been lonely since their husbands worked outside the home for long periods of time; they were no longer closely attached to their extended families; they were isolated in the suburbs; there were fewer opportunities to participate in community and civic events; and the majority of mothers had become highly dependent upon the expertise of child-rearing experts to rear their children. In summary, women had already lost true dominion over the privacy of family life many decades earlier.

Despite these and many other reasons for women's lack of fulfillment, the one objective of encouraging women to work outside the home has been proclaimed to be the panacea for women who felt as frustrated and unhappy as did the mothers of Conway, Reichl, and Roiphe. The supposition is that these wives and mothers should have had the opportunity to do something more meaningful with their lives. Consequently, an obsessive focus has been placed upon addressing the needs of women as if they do not become wives and mothers.

The feminist agenda, as discussed earlier, links a women's self-identity inextricably to the work she does outside the home. Although the persistent presence of women in the workforce is an important and sensible objective for women as a whole, it is not necessarily either reasonable or merciful for mothers of young children. Had these women had the opportunity to work outside the home, it is assumed that they might have been more content, and they would have had no need to wreak havoc on their daughters' lives. Or as many feminists would argue today, women who work outside the home are more fulfilled personally and, therefore, are better mothers. Is this true, though?

One should wonder why the happiness and self-identity of a woman should be attached so definitively to her employment outside the home. Why is this any healthier or better than having a woman's identity secured to being a fulfilled mother to her children? Ultimately, encouraging or even demanding women's fealty to work outside the home will turn out to be confounding because there is nothing inherently stable about identifying one's happiness or self-identity with one's employment. The work arenas into which women have entered in recent decades are the same ones that have long employed men.

The modern workplace is centered upon work ethics that have clearly lost their humanity. Life-long employment and guaranteed pensions at major corporations, which once provided job security for countless blue-collar and white-collar employees, are no longer part of the American business plan. The longevity of the small business owners who once buttressed entire communities is passé as huge companies have entered even the smallest markets. Important entry level jobs that once provided future advancement in fields like banking, accounting, and telecommunications are now being outsourced abroad to countries where the English language is spoken, and employees earn significantly lower wages. Essentially, no American job today offers security similar to that which was offered to a wide array of workers a mere generation ago.

This subject was addressed in an article in an April 2003 issue of the *New York Times Magazine*. It features three male executives, their struggles with unemployment, and their attempts to gain new employment. The three men were all once successful and highly paid white-collar employees who lost their jobs after the U.S. economy started to weaken in 2000. Although the three men face their travails valiantly, the saddest portrayal is that of the executive who winds up working at the Gap clothing store even though he once earned $300,000 per year. He is unable to secure a high-paying job, and various financial investments have not worked in his favor. His stress is compounded by his wife's disappointment and anger at having become the family's primary breadwinner.

Although employees may seek stability in their work life, the current work world offers few or no guarantees of security or loyalty to any employee. Ultimately, complete devotion to work life may not necessarily offer consequential security to any employee, regardless of gender or socioeconomic background. In a volatile work environment that treats employees as if they are dispensable, both women and men face unstable employment conditions. It is in this unstable work world, however, that a woman is supposed to find and maintain her true self-identity.

Over the last several decades, feminists have made significant strides by gaining women greater and more equal access to higher education and employment. They have achieved this, however, at the expense of ignoring a woman's identity as a wife and mother. What is truly worrisome is that a woman's responsibility in caring for her children has become so irrelevant to the feminist agenda that it is becoming tolerable for women to express indifference to their children's well-being.

THE APATHETIC MOTHER

There are women and men who can apparently state with frank honesty that they do not appreciate the value of family life. For example, the content and proud mother of a 34-year-old man told me recently that other women have told her that they regret having become mothers. The possibility that a woman might regret having become a mother is not new. What is surprising, however, is the extent to which such an attitude has become less stigmatized. Divorce and consecutive marriages have become culturally acceptable over the past few decades, and soon it will become similarly unobjectionable for a woman to become apathetic to the fate of her child.

The prevailing sentiment seems to be that if individuals are dissatisfied with their families, it is all right to abandon them and start anew elsewhere without them. Hence, there are novels like Anne Tyler's *Ladder of Years*, which seem to infer that abandonment can actually be an eye-opening experience that improves family life. Ultimately, Tyler is optimistic in her outlook on family life since she still trusts that it has some meaning. What happens, though, when family life and maternal love lose all meaning, and a woman possesses a passion to satisfy only her needs and desires?

An extreme depiction of such a woman was offered by Edith Wharton in her novel *The Custom of the Country*, which was published originally in 1913. Undine Spragg, the protagonist of the novel, is a beautiful, ambitious, and utterly self-centered creature who seeks to be glorified and adulated by high society. She believes that she can gain access to the highest reaches of New York society by marrying Ralph Marvell, an upper-class but fairly impoverished New Yorker.

Undine is terribly extravagant, vain, inconsiderate, and manipulative. When she becomes pregnant, her gentle and loving husband pleads with her to see the bright side of pregnancy. She retorts angrily, "It takes a year—a whole year out of life! What do I care how I shall feel in a year?" (Wharton 2001, 114). After Undine gives birth, she promptly abandons her newborn to the care of a nanny, Ralph, and Ralph's mother and sister.

Undine is an indifferent mother and an unloving wife: she embarks on an illicit affair with a wealthy cad, eventually divorces Ralph and abandons her baby, and marries twice more. Her unscrupulous ways sadly precipitate Ralph's tragic demise and force her son to leave his beloved aunt and grandmother. By the time Undine's son, Paul, is nine years old, he has experienced far too much suffering as a result of his mother's caprices.

Undine has disrupted Paul's ties to the Marvell family as well as those the boy had established with her second ex-husband. Meanwhile, she remains oblivious to her son's need for maternal affection and attention. When he tries to hug her one day, she rebuffs him and exclaims, "Gracious, how you squeeze!" She then leaves him as he tries to tell her that he has won a prize in composition. Undine's new husband, Mr. Moffatt, sympathizes with the distraught and crying boy. He attempts to bolster the boy's spirits and says, "Is it because your mother hadn't time for you? Well, she's like that, you know; and you and I have got to lump it" (2001, 360).

Undine is preoccupied since she is about to entertain prominent guests whose respect she has been seeking since her first introduction to high society. Her sentiments are summed up as follows: "Even now, however, she was not always happy. She had everything she wanted, but she still felt, at times, that there were other things she might want if she knew about them. And there had been moments lately when she had had to confess to herself that Moffatt did not fit into the picture" (2001, 362–363). Undine is dissatisfied even though she has fulfilled her aspirations of attaining incredible wealth, status, and power. Undine's priorities were and always will be self-centered, for she was reared to be like this by her indulgent parents and by the American culture that promoted such behavior.

Edith Wharton's indictment of high society at the turn of the twentieth century is significant because it exposes the demeaned type of existence wealthier Americans were already leading a century ago. At the heart of unhappy family life often lay the inexorable demands of work life made upon men to support lavish lifestyles for their wives. One of the novel's characters, an astute social observer named Charles Bowen decries how the hard-working husband often refuses to share with his wife the difficulties he faces at work. Bowen argues that when women remain purposefully ignorant of work life, they concentrate their lives on frivolous aspects of life related to consumerism and their appearance.

Bowen calls this "the custom of the country," wherein men are completely absorbed in the domain of work whereas women are wholly excluded. Bowen assesses a creature like Undine Spragg to be the product of such a custom, describing her as the "monstrously perfect result of the system: the completest proof of its triumph" (2001, 128). Undine is no more interested in her various husbands' work than she is with the work of caring for her own child and the maintenance of her home. Work, as she understands it, is merely the domain of her father and her husbands who must provide her with the funds to pursue her interests and ambition.

Undine Spragg is precisely the type of woman whom early feminists considered not to be useful to society. Educated to become shallow and parasitic, Undine is the antithesis of intelligent and capable women who wished to make worthwhile contributions to society by working outside the home. Paradoxically, women like Undine and early feminists were more similar than they either knew or would have admitted: both groups of women were more concerned with the satisfaction of womanly ambition outside the home than they were with the fulfillment of the maternal role inside the home.

REPLACING MOTHERS

Fundamentally, feminists have been as self-centered as Undine Spragg in the way they have disregarded the importance of child-rearing and family life. Charlotte Perkins Gilman, for instance, embraced work life and thought family life presented terrible restrictions on women's freedom. Gilman (1983, 395) even proposed communal kitchens in order to eliminate the need for individual families to cook in the home: "The performance of domestic industries involves, first, an enormous waste of labor.... We pay rent for twenty kitchens where one kitchen would do." The line of reasoning was that if family-related chores could be obviated, then women could participate in meaningful work life outside the home.

From this type of thinking arose the idea that child care could become a cooperative effort that did not need to be centered upon family life. The women's movement, as noted earlier in Chapter 13, has always prioritized work life over family life and the care of children. This mind-set, ironically, was not much different from that of Undine, who preferred the tasks of beautifying herself and socializing over the work of caring for her son and husbands. Needless to say, feminists' objectives were nobler, like getting women to excel in the arts and sciences, but one should not overlook the deliberate way in which feminists have disregarded the significance of child-rearing.

If the majority of women had chosen to follow the feminist agenda, then they would have remained childless, and the conflict between work life and family life would not have arisen to the magnitude it has today. If anything, feminists would have realized their dream of gaining true equality for women in society. The troubling reality, however, is that the majority of women have continued to bear children who need to be reared.

Women may have wanted to follow the feminist agenda and gain access to meaningful work outside the home, but the majority also wanted to have a family life. Consequently, the majority of women now face the dilemma of caring for their young children and wanting or needing to return to work outside the home. As women are encouraged to pursue their occupations and personal ambitions outside the home, few consider how young children will fare in the absence of maternal care.

Feminists advocate universal day care as being the only viable option for child-rearing since they assume that women should work outside the home in order to support a relatively high standard of living. There is merit to the argument that high quality day care may enable talented and capable mothers to work outside the home. Increasingly, large corporations and non-profit institutions are creating on-site day care centers that permit women to work outside the home while remaining near their young babies and toddlers.

On a personal note I have friends who work outside the home while their children attend high quality day care centers run by their employers. For instance, one friend took an extended maternity leave and then placed her son in a day care center adjacent to her workplace. She managed to nurse her son several times a day and was able to maintain a prolonged breastfeeding relationship with her son through his toddler years. She now has a second son in the same day care center, and she is able to nurse him frequently as well. Although both young children are in day care, my friend notices that they enjoy good health and intimacy with her and her husband because of prolonged breastfeeding.

Another friend holds a prominent academic position at a prestigious medical school. From early infancy, her two children have been in a day care center that is affiliated with the medical school. She was also able to breastfeed her two babies. An annual Christmas photograph of the family depicts a happy and thriving family.

The success of my friends is what feminists understandably applaud with great vigor. Both of my friends placed their children in high quality day care centers while they worked outside the home and contributed to society. The reality, though, is that my friends were fortunate since, as mentioned earlier in Chapter 10, only one in seven day care centers offers young babies and children excellent care. In other words, the chances of finding excellent day care for one's child are low.

There are now millions of babies and young children who are surviving and supposedly thriving in the absence of consistent maternal care. Advocates of day care cite repeatedly research that purports to show that young children might become more socially adept and better students if they are put in day care instead of home care. The underlying premise is that educated professionals can provide stimulating care that would enable young children to learn more at an earlier age. These ambitious early childhood education goals are mentioned despite the fact that there are few day care centers that can provide young children with such high quality professional care in the U.S.

In the meantime, there is no proof that learning more at an earlier age necessarily predicts children's future success either socially or academically. Additionally, there are many cases in which brilliant and seemingly promising young children mature into delinquents, criminals, or mentally ill adults. Even so, the push for universal day care remains forceful and unrelenting whereas the possibility of providing more youngsters with the benefits of maternal care is not even considered.

Several years ago, advocates of universal day care in the U.S. expressed overt interest in the government-sponsored day care and pre-school systems that are available in France. Babies from six months to three years of age may be enrolled in a crèche, a high quality day care center, at a cost to parents of approximately

$10 per day (French-American Foundation 2005). From the age of two years, as long as the child is toilet trained, all children living in France are eligible to attend pre-school, or école maternelle, free of cost (Peer, Baudelot, and Neuman 2004). Attendance is nearly universal for the highly regarded and respected day care and pre-school systems in France because these teachers are trained well, and they are regarded highly.

Undoubtedly, French parents trust that the care and education their young babies and children receive in the crèche and école maternelle will enhance their growth and development. Nevertheless, despite the widespread availability of such high quality day care, French school-aged children have been exhibiting undisciplined, aggressive, and violent behavior. A 1998 article in *Mother Jones* reports that French adolescents were inciting riots and perpetrating violence against police officers, fire fighters, bus drivers, and elderly bystanders. French authorities associate the rise in juvenile crime to the violence children see in movies and video games, as well as on television. The French Education Minister "pledged thousands of additional staff, more police and toughened sanctions against students as part of new measures to curb mounting violence in schools" (The Tocqueville Connection 2000).

The reports of increased violence among French children indicate that irrespective of the widespread availability of seemingly ideal, highly professional, and affordable or free day care and early education in France, something is seriously amiss with current French child-rearing practices. There are no signs of significant or visible improvement in the condition of these children's humanity. If anything, there has been a precipitous decline in civility and cooperative behavior.

From many perspectives, it appears that access to high quality day care and excellent pre-school educational preparation may be highly desirable. This is especially relevant for the children of working class women. It is obvious, however, that the majority of children do not benefit by receiving non-maternal care on a full-time basis from early infancy.

Again, the real question that should be asked is not even addressed: Is maternal care truly dispensable? The reason this question is not even brought up is that it is assumed de facto that mothers can no longer afford not to work outside the home. The value of maternal care, however, should not be underestimated. Mothers make invaluable contributions to society by rearing fulfilled children who will mature into healthy, civil, and cooperative adults.

It is absurd to continue to misunderstand the importance of maternal care in a child's life. Just as Anne Roiphe admits that her writing reverts constantly to the recollection of her need to be near her unaware mother, the most primary desire of a young child is to be with a loving mother. To deny the importance of maternal care is equivalent to denying one's humanity which, unfortunately, can be done all too easily.

FORGING LOVE

Even though parents may wish to be more emotionally connected and communicative with their children, many work long hours outside the home. The lack of consistent parental availability plays a significant role in interfering with the development of a healthy and loving relationship between parents and children since love is nurtured through hard work, effort, and availability. Plainly stated, it is difficult for parents and children to establish a mutually loving relationship when parents are simply unavailable.

Parents are assured, however, that a mother's presence in the home is unnecessary and that both parents' quest for self-fulfillment and productivity at work outside the home will not affect adversely their children's development and growth. These assurances are given despite the precarious nature of such assumptions. The reality is that it is farcical to presume that the love between parents and children can maintain its own force and vitality when children do not receive consistent parental love.

Current child-rearing practices constitute a broad social experiment that blatantly ignores the most fundamental and unique relationship in the history of humankind: the mother-child relationship. It is almost wishful thinking to trust that children will thrive in an environment that excludes a loving and available mother, but this has become a standard child-rearing practice. It is widely and inexplicably assumed that babies and children will become healthy adults as long as they are provided with rudimentary care. Who is to say, however, that today's young babies and children will turn out to be socialized and compassionate adults in the future?

In recent years it has even become acceptable to regard a child's survival to be subordinate to that of his mother. This is, in effect, the opinion of the actress Julianne Moore, who portrays the fictional character of Laura Brown in the film version of *The Hours.* When a *Newsweek* journalist in December 2002 asks Moore about the character's deserted husband and children, she dismisses the inquiry as being irrelevant. Moore asserts that the integrity of the role lies in Laura Brown's ability to prioritize her needs before those of others. Moore's point is that women should embrace selfishness and disregard altruism even when the well-being of one's spouse and children are at risk.

In other words, it has become fashionable to suggest that one should seek out good primarily for oneself. Who is to say, however, that such selfish survival is either a healthy or good way of life? There are real consequences to self-centered behavior, and they can be destructive and harmful to others, particularly loved ones. One hardly expects selfish behavior from a mother, but it has become commonplace for women to assert the primacy of their need for independence and self-fulfillment.

Nearly a century ago, Virginia Woolf offered a contrasting portrayal of a woman who exudes greatness and power in the maternal role. Her novel *To the Lighthouse* depicts the amazing character of Mrs. Ramsay, a beloved mother and wife. Mrs. Ramsay is a woman upon whom everyone depends for her beauty, grace, goodness, love, trustworthiness, compassion, and genuine concern. Her positive attributes do not arise from nothing or by chance: they are the fruits of a state of being, one that is based upon altruism and the willingness to make efforts on behalf of others.

This novel affirms the tremendous power of women and the profoundly positive impact their love and hard work has upon their family life and community. Mrs. Ramsay affects everyone around her greatly. One of the characters, the artist Lily Briscoe, returns to the seaside and recalls her experiences with Mrs. Ramsay. Lily has been unable to complete a painting for years, but in a single moment, she is able to draw a line down the center of the canvas, and her painting is done. With that scene, Virginia Woolf describes the power that exists within one's life to either create art as Lily does or nurture life as Mrs. Ramsay does.

The novel also describes how little human beings know one another, even if they have been married for a long time. For example, Mrs. Ramsay looks at her husband one day and wonders how little she knows him. It is almost irrelevant since they have lived together for many years, and each is fully aware of the other's strengths and weaknesses. Woolf (1927, 123–124) describes how Mr. and Mrs. Ramsay sometimes interact with one another:

> And what then? For she felt that he was still looking at her, but that his look had changed. He wanted something—wanted the thing she always found it so difficult to give him; wanted her to tell him that she loved him. And that, no, she could not do. He found talking so much easier than she did.... Then, knowing that he was watching her, instead of saying anything she turned, holding her stocking, and looked at him. And as she looked at him she began to smile, for though she had not said a word, he knew, of course he knew, that

> she loved him. He could not deny it. And smiling she looked out of the window and said (thinking to herself, Nothing on earth can equal this happiness)—.

Naturally, it is impossible to delve into the depths of anyone else's mind, but one tries with loved ones. One appreciates the love that can be shared despite the vast differences in the personality and behavior of the various members of a family. It is worth the effort to fight for and win such love regardless of the hardships involved in maintaining family life, however imperfect it may be.

My interpretation of Mrs. Ramsay's character may be contested by others who have read *To the Lighthouse*. Other readers might perceive that the novel portrays an indictment of family life rather than an embrace of it. In reality, there is nothing perfect about the life Mrs. Ramsay leads. Her children are unhappy often enough, and there is frequent discord between Mr. and Mrs. Ramsay. Nevertheless, the force of Mrs. Ramsay's life and her efforts sustain and draw the family together.

RESPECTING MOTHERS

It takes talent and strength to be the pillar of a family and provide the succor that family members need so frequently. In many ways, Mrs. Ramsay is imperfect as a loving wife and mother; she even admits that she has difficulty expressing her love. Even so, Mrs. Ramsay's existence revolves around giving to and sharing with others, a feat she manages by restoring her own sense of self constantly.

At the end of each day, Mrs. Ramsay knits as she sits in her rocking chair and looks out toward the lighthouse. She is in a transcendent state, and she imagines that she is traveling far away to different lands. As she is absorbed in this state of being, she draws energy from the strength of her imagination and the light that emanates from the lighthouse. During this time, however brief it may be, she rests and rejuvenates herself. It is Mrs. Ramsay's opportunity to spend some moments alone and undisturbed, away from family members who expect and receive so much from her. This period of self-reflection seems to give Mrs. Ramsay spiritual strength.

The hope for women today is that they can replenish their life force as they nurture their family life despite the myriad directions in which their lives are pulled. The stresses of living in modern society are numerous, but the quest to provide young children with the nurturing they deserve should still be the foremost priority. No matter how difficult life may be, the efforts that women make toward the creation of a consequential family life are irreplaceable and invaluable.

Surely, many families can argue justifiably that they are doing their utmost to create a consequential family life. Undoubtedly, this is true since many parents are working harder than ever to maintain a lifestyle that seems comparable to that of their parents. It must nevertheless be acknowledged that the modern lifestyle is nothing like the average middle-class lifestyle of even a generation ago.

In the modern era, make-work reigns, and money must be earned in order for families to purchase as many goods as possible. Accordingly, women pursue work and income outside the home while leaving their young children in the care of others. Although it may be true that families are doing their best for their children, there is little doubt that the true value of hands-on maternal care is underestimated persistently and unabashedly.

In the 2003 comedy film *Head of State*, comedian and actor Chris Rock portrays a presidential candidate who decries the fact that women no longer care for their own babies. His campaign slogan is: "That ain't right!" In a scene at a day care center, the candidate holds a young child in his lap and describes the conundrum of modern child-rearing practices: a working mother takes her child to a nanny; the nanny takes her child to a babysitter; and the babysitter takes her child to a day care. Then he offers the following suggestion: "Now, on the count of three, I want everybody to take care of your own damn kids!"

Mothering is an art that has to be learned. The prevailing assumption may be that mothering is expendable, but it is not. Mothering is an art that improves with practice, patience, dedication, and love. It is time for contemporary society to learn how to respect mothers and the unique and irreplaceable role they play in children's lives, family life, and society.

APPENDIX A

WHAT IS BREAST MILK?

COLOSTRUM

Colostrum is a thick, yellowish fluid that a mother's breasts produce in small quantities. It is enriched with protein, fat soluble vitamins (A, E, and carotenoids which give the colostrum the characteristic yellow color), and minerals. Colostrum plays a crucial role in providing breastfed infants with immunological protection since it is rich in immunoglobulins, which are antibodies that provide both passive and active immunity against various pathogens.

Colostrum contains high levels of Secretory IgA, an immunoglobulin that has been shown to provide important intestinal protection for young infants against viruses and bacteria. Secretory IgA protects infants against poliovirus and harmful bacteria like E. coli (a major cause of diarrheal illnesses), Staphylococcus, and even some fungi. Colostrum also contains live white blood cells that can ingest germs.

Colostrum provides the infant's immature digestive tract with the correct stimuli for healthy gut development. It contains a specific factor that supports the growth of Lactobacillus bifidus which are gram-positive, anaerobic, nonmotile rod shaped bacteria. Bifid bacteria are beneficial bacteria that predominate in the intestinal tracts of breastfed babies.

Colostrum is also a potent laxative that serves to clear the newborn's gut of the sticky black stool called meconium. Clearing of the meconium from the gut helps to decrease both the incidence and severity of jaundice, the yellowing of the skin and sclerae of the eyes. Very importantly, the small amounts of potent colostrum that are secreted for the first seven to ten days after birth complement the needs of an immature neonatal digestive tract.

In *Milk, Money, and Madness*, Naomi Baumslag and Dia Michels (1995, 74) write, "Colostrum contains many of the same antibodies and nutrients found in mature milk, but in a concentrated form, making it the ultimate food at a time when the baby is extremely vulnerable yet has low caloric needs." The high protein content of colostrum is thought to stabilize the newborn's blood sugar.

Within the first week of life, it is normal for a newborn to lose up to ten percent of her body weight. An exclusively breastfed baby who suckles consistently at the breast will stimulate the production of greater volumes of milk. A healthy baby will regain her weight naturally by breastfeeding exclusively. Although initial breastfeeding sessions may yield only two teaspoons of colostrum, by two weeks of age most babies are drinking from twenty-eight to thirty-two ounces of breast milk per day (1995, 75).

INCOMPARABLE BREAST MILK

After colostrum, a mother's breasts produce transitional milk from about seven to ten days after birth to two weeks after birth. The protein concentration decreases, as does the immunoglobulin concentration. On the other hand, the fat, lactose, and total caloric content will increase.

The levels of fat soluble vitamins decrease while the water soluble vitamins increase. With the production of transitional milk, a breastfed baby will begin to gain weight that was lost during the first week of life. By approximately two weeks after birth, a breastfeeding baby will be suckling mature milk.

Breastfeeding researcher Ruth Lawrence devotes a lengthy chapter in *Breastfeeding: A Guide for the Medical Profession* to the many components in human milk that offer breastfed infants immunological protection. Neonates are at high risk for bacterial infection after birth because they are born immunologically immature despite having received some protection from the placenta. Dr. Lawrence (1999, 160) writes, "The newborn cannot muster the same level of defense against infection that an adult is capable of developing."

After birth, the newborn should ingest colostrum that is rich in live cells and able to help in fighting infection. In countries as diverse as Pakistan and Sweden, breastfeeding has been shown to reduce the incidence of infection in the newborn. Overall, breastfed babies have a much lower incidence of diarrheal disease, respiratory infections, and ear infections.

Naomi Baumslag and Dia Michels (1995, 84–87) also detail how different human milk is from cow's milk. Compared to cow's milk, human milk contains:

- higher levels of cholesterol, used in brain tissue development and myelinization of nerves;

- higher levels of polyunsaturated fatty acids, particularly linoleic acid; deficiencies have been associated with the development of skin lesions, growth retardation, and poor wound healing;
- higher levels of whey as compared with curds, making human milk more easily digestible, and thus explaining breastfed infants' need to nurse frequently;
- cysteine, an essential amino acid; cow's milk has methionine, instead of cysteine, which cannot be metabolized by the human infant's immature liver;
- the whey proteins lactalbumin and lactoferrin; lactoferrin is thought to bind the iron in germs that cause gastrointestinal infections, thereby stopping their infectious action in the infant's gut; cow's milk contains primarily betalactoglobulin, not lactoferrin;
- lactose delivered in constant amounts; it provides glucose and galactose, which are both important for the development of nervous tissue; it is also an instant source of energy and it aids in the absorption of calcium;
- zinc that is efficiently absorbed; Acrodermatitis enteropathica, a deficiency in zinc, is found only in formula-fed infants and can be cured with breast milk or zinc supplementation;
- vitamin C which is efficiently absorbed as long as a mother's diet contains adequate amounts of Vitamin C; formula-fed babies need Vitamin C supplements;
- high levels of Vitamins D, E, and K, particularly in colostrum, and high levels of Vitamin A and folic acid as long as a mother's diet is adequate; most pediatricians recommend a supplement of Vitamin K after birth to prevent late onset of hemorrhagic disease associated with Vitamin K deficiency;
- low levels of iron because of excellent iron absorption; in contrast, infant formula contains very high levels of iron that interfere with the anti-infectious properties of lactoferrin, possibly leading to a greater risk of infection.

Breast milk consists of numerous different elements that work together in many ways to provide the human infant and toddler with the ability to fight infection. Both colostrum and human milk contain live white blood cells such as macrophages and lymphocytes. Macrophages can eat fungi and bacteria, kill bacteria, and possibly store lymphocytes. Lymphocytes have been found to react against germs that invade the gut.

Breast milk also contains immunoglobulins, of which IgA appears to play an important role in fighting infection. Specific antibodies to the harmful bacteria *E. coli* persist through breastfeeding. Antibodies in breast milk kill polio virus, cholera, the giardia parasite, and some fungi (Baumslag and Michels 1995, 89). A resistance factor has been identified in human milk that protects the breastfed infant against staphylococcal bacterial infection.

Lysozyme is an enzyme that can help to break down the cell walls of some bacteria, thus preventing further bacterial growth. Lactoferrin binds iron so that iron is unavailable for use by iron-dependent germs, including some bacteria and yeast. An interferon-like substance in human milk has anti-viral activity. There are numerous other substances in breast milk that work in conjunction with each other to provide the breastfed infant and child enormous protection from infection.

Breast milk itself is a complex and dynamic liquid that contains numerous other components that function in diverse ways. Dr. Lawrence devotes a chapter in her textbook on breastfeeding to the biochemistry of human milk. The following is a brief summary of how some of the components of human milk function:

- amylase may inhibit growth of certain microorganisms;
- lipases break down fats to free fatty acids, making human milk more digestible;
- lactose synthetase catalyzes the formation of lactose;
- lysozyme catalyzes the breakdown of certain bacterial cell walls, plays a role in antibacterial activity of human milk, and helps to break down mucopolysaccharides;
- proteases provide significant digestive assistance immediately after birth;
- anti-proteases may protect the mammary gland and the infant from infection and help to transfer immunoglobulins intact to the infant;
- thyroid hormone can protect infants who have a deficiency in thyroid hormone;
- prostaglandins may play a role in gastrointestinal motility and the enhancement of the gastric mucosal barrier;
- bile salts are thought to contribute to the newborn's digestion;

- epidermal growth factor is thought to be a major growth-promoting agent in breast milk (Lawrence 1999, 144–149).

Oligosaccharides in breast milk are sugars with special receptors that are similar to receptors in the infant's intestinal cells (Newman and Pittman 2000, 275). Bacteria may bind to the oligosaccharides instead of the infant's intestinal cells. Instead of causing infection, the bacteria are eliminated in the baby's bowel movement.

In conclusion, breast milk contains a vast array of important and crucial substances that help to determine the healthy growth and development of babies. There is simply no comparison between breastfeeding and the use of infant formula. Additionally, there are many more substances in human milk that either have not yet been identified or whose role has not yet been clarified.

APPENDIX B

SUCKLING AT THE BREAST

The following is a summary of Ashley Montagu's description of suckling (1986, 82–6):

1. There is a short critical period for the establishment of the suckling reflex. Thus, it is important for the newborn to suckle at the breast as soon as possible after birth.

2. The baby draws the entire areola (darkened tissue around the nipple) into his mouth because the suckling reflex is triggered off by stimulation of the lips and touch receptors deep in the mouth.

3. The baby suckles not on the nipple, a common misperception, but the areolar region. The collecting sinuses, located under the areola, are pressed by the baby's lips and gums to express the milk.

4. The nipple is drawn to the back of the mouth. It is compressed between the upper gum and the tip of the tongue, which rests on the lower gum. The tongue is applied to the lower surface of the nipple and drawn backwards while compressing it against the hard palate.

5. Suckling induces the secretion of two pituitary hormones, prolactin and oxytocin. Prolactin is responsible for the maintenance of milk secretion. Oxytocin is concerned with the milk ejection or the "letdown" reflex.

6. The nipple and areola are drawn into the mouth and sealed by lips and the buccinator muscles. The lips are highly sensitive to touch and the upper lip is equipped with a median papilla (the little protrusion in the middle of the upper lip) that ensures a firm grip on the areola.

7. The areola has a roughened surface, caused by numerous elevations produced by the underlying areolar glands. They secrete fatty material that lubricates and protects the areola and nipple during nursing.

8. The suctorial pads located in the baby's cheeks, giving them their rounded form, are primarily responsible for setting up the negative pressure that draws the milk into the oral cavity.

9. Most babies have a narrow fold of erectile tissue at the base of the outer side of the gum called Magitot's membrane. During suckling, this membrane becomes quite swollen and assists in tightly sealing the areola in the mouth. This membrane usually disappears by six months of age.

10. A baby presses his jaws and face against his mother's breast, first at one breast and then at the other. Thus, both sides of the face, jaws, and other parts of the body receive a great deal of stimulation that is denied to the bottle-fed baby who is usually held in the same position for feedings.

APPENDIX C

CONTRAINDICATIONS TO BREASTFEEDING

Breastfeeding is the optimal way to nourish young children for the first year of life. According to the American Academy of Pediatrics (AAP) Policy Statement on Breastfeeding (2005), there are a few situations in which breastfeeding is not recommended. As an experienced pediatrician who has studied breastfeeding extensively, Dr. Jack Newman offers a different perspective on some of these recommendations.

Dr. Newman also recommends that physicians and breastfeeding mothers use a textbook by pharmacologist Dr. Thomas Hale called *Medications and Mother's Milk*, published by Pharmasoft Medical Publishing and updated every two years. It clarifies when mothers who are taking medications should stop breastfeeding, and it also includes recommendations for alternative medications that are compatible with breastfeeding.

The following are situations in which the AAP does not recommend breastfeeding, and Dr. Newman's suggestions are added:

- Infants with classic galactosemia (deficiency in the enzyme galactose 1-phosphate uridyltransferase). The galactose in lactose cannot be metabolized, and its build-up is dangerous for the infant. The incidence of this rare disease is 1 out of 600,000 live births. Dr. Newman (2000, 173) agrees that this is one of the few true medical reasons to stop breastfeeding.

- Mothers who have active tuberculosis disease. Dr. Newman (287–288) assesses that the most important step that needs to be taken is immediate medical treatment for the mother. The breast milk itself is not infectious. If the mother's sputum is positive for the infectious germ, he recommends that breastfeeding not be stopped as long as the mother is being treated with medication, and she wears a surgical mask to prevent spreading contagious germs from her lungs and sputum. The baby should be given BCG, a vaccine against tuberculosis, and treated with an anti-tuberculosis medication like Isoniazid.

- Mothers who are receiving diagnostic or therapeutic radioactive isotopes or have had exposure to radioactive materials (for as long as there is radioactivity in the milk). The most commonly used radioactive compound for studies is technetium 99, which has a half-life of 6 hours and should be cleared from the mother's body after 30 hours. Dr. Newman (266) assesses this to be a long period of time that may be unnecessary. He questions the need to wait until the breast milk is cleared of all radioactive material since infants may themselves receive diagnostic tests with the same radioactive material. In the case of radioactive iodine that is used for thyroid scans, the long half-life of over 13 hours poses a problem for the breastfeeding mother in that she would need to stop breastfeeding for over 65 hours. Dr. Newman (267) questions the need for the use of radioactive iodine and argues that the scan may be done with technetium 99.
- Mothers who are receiving antimetabolites or chemotherapeutic agents.
- Mothers who are using illicit drugs or "street drugs." No one advocates the use of illicit drugs, but there are numerous individuals, including breastfeeding mothers, who may indulge in such habits. Dr. Newman (263) opines that the occasional use of marijuana should not interfere with breastfeeding, but excessive use of marijuana will concentrate the active ingredient, THC, in the milk and its effects on the nursling are unknown. The use of illicit drugs benefits neither the mother nor the nursling, and such behavior needs to be stopped. Breastfeeding, from Dr. Newman's perspective (264) may help a mother boost her self-esteem and enable her to care better for her infant and herself.
- Mothers who have herpes simplex lesions on a breast may permit the baby to nurse on the other breast. Active lesions can be contagious, and it would be best for the baby to avoid contact with the lesions.
- Mothers in the U.S. who are infected with HIV (Human Immune Deficiency Virus) are advised not to breastfeed. Please see Chapter 8, Myth # 8 for more information.

WORKS CITED

Abramson, Jill, and Barbara Franklin. 1986. *Where they are now*. New York: Doubleday.

Al-Azzawi, Farook. 1990. *Childbirth and obstetric techniques*. New York: Mosby Year Book.

American Academy of Pediatrics (AAP). 2003. Policy statement: Prevention of pediatric overweight and obesity. *Pediatrics* 112 (August): 424–430.

———. 2005. Policy statement: Breastfeeding and the use of human milk. *Pediatrics* 115 (February): 496–506.

American Council on Education. 2000. ACE study shows gains in number of women college presidents, smaller gains for minority CEOs. September 11. http://www.acenet.edu/news/press_release/2000/09september/college-president.html.

American Demographics. 2002. The baby sabbatical-statistical data included. February 1. http://www.findarticles.com/p/articles/mi_m4021/is_2002_Feb_1/ai_82264577.

Anand, KJS, and International Evidence-Based Group for Neonatal Pain. 2001. Consensus statement for the prevention and management of pain in the newborn. *Archives of Pediatric and Adolescent Medicine* 155(2):173–180.

Apple, Rima D. 1987. *Mothers and medicine: A social history of infant feeding 1890–1950*. Madison, WI: The University of Wisconsin Press.

Atkinson, Robert D. 2003. Putting parenting first: Why it's time for universal paid leave. Progressive Policy Institute. March. http://www.ppionline.org/ppi_ci.cfm?contentid=251419&subsecid=144&knlgAreaID=114

Baker, S. Josephine. 1992. Fighting for life. In *Written by herself: Volume I.: Autobiographies of American women: An anthology.* Ed. Jill Ker Conway. New York: Vintage Books.

Barad, David. 2004. Age and female fertility. American Fertility Association. http://www.theafa.org/faqs/afa_ageandfemaleinfertility.html.

Baumslag, Naomi, and Dia Michels. 1995. *Milk, money, and madness.* Westport, CT: Bergin and Garvey.

Blum, Deborah. 2002. *Love at Goon Park: Harry Harlow and the science of affection.* Cambridge: Perseus Publishing.

Boorstin, Daniel J. 1985. *The discoverers: A history of man's search to know his world and himself.* New York: Vintage Books.

Boykin, Cynthia, and Dennis Harper. 2004. Depression in children and adolescents. Virtual Children's Hospital. http://www.vh.org/pediatric/provider/pediatrics/depression/.

Brenna, J. Thomas. 2003. Infant formulas containing DHA and ARA. Cornell Cooperative Extension. April 4. http://www.cce.cornell.edu/food/expfiles/topics/brenna/brennaoverview.html.

California Department of Health Services. 2005. California WIC breastfeeding mission statement. http://www.wicworks.ca.gov/breastfeeding/downloads/Mission%20Statement%20English%20and%20Spanish%20%20Final.pdf.

Caplan, Mariana. 1998. *Untouched: The need for genuine affection in an impersonal world.* Prescott, AZ: Hohm Press.

Centers for Disease Control and Prevention (CDC). 1995. Rates of cesarean delivery—United States, 1993. Morbidity and Mortality Weekly Report (MMWR). April 21. http://www.cdc.gov/mmwr/preview/mmwrhtml/00036845.htm.

———. 2004a. Birth rate for women aged 40–44 years rose in 2003, new report finds. National Center for Health Statistics. November 23. http://www.cdc.gov/nchs/pressroom/04facts/birthrates.htm.

———. 2004b. Chronology of significant developments related to smoking and health. Tobacco Information and Prevention Source (TIPS). May 2. http://www.cdc.gov/tobacco/overview/chron96.htm.

———. 2004c. Overweight and obese: Frequently asked questions. October 20. http://www.cdc.gov/nccdphp/dnpa/obesity/faq.htm.

Cesarean Childbirth. 2005. eMedicine Consumer Health. April 6. http://www.emedicinehealth.com/articles/12168-1.asp

Cheever, Susan. 1995. The nanny track. *New Yorker,* March 6.

Conway, Jill Ker. 1989. *The road from Coorain.* New York: Vintage Books.

Coutsoudis, Anna. 2005. Current status of HIV and breastfeeding research. *Breastfeeding Abstracts* 24 (February): 11–12.

Cunningham, Michael. 1998. *The hours.* New York: Picador U.S.A.

Dermer, Alicia, and Anne Montgomery. 1997. Breastfeeding: Good for babies, mothers, and the planet. *The Medical Reporter* II (11). http://medicalreporter.health.org/tmr0297/breastfeed0297.html.

Dettwyler, Katherine. 1995. A time to wean: The hominid blueprint for the natural age of weaning in modern human populations. In *Breastfeeding: Biocultural perspectives.* Eds. Patricia Stuart-Macadam and Katherine A. Dettwyler. New York: Aldine de Gruyter.

Drugs.com. 1997. Bromocriptine (systemic). Drug Information Online. August 20. http://www.drugs.com/MMX/Bromocriptine_Mesylate.html.

Finch, Cristin, and Eileen Daniel. 2002. A breastfeeding education program-breastfeeding and prenatal nutrition issues. *Nutrition Research Letter.* August. http://www.google.com/search?hl=en&q=breastfeeding+among+WIC+participans.

Food and Drug Administration (FDA). 2003. Infant formula: Frequently asked questions. U.S. Food and Drug Administration. U.S. Department of Health and Human Services. January 9. http://www.cfsan.fda.gov/~dms/qa-inf21.html.

Fox, Isabelle. 1996. *Being there: The benefits of a stay-at-home parent.* Hauppage, NY: Barron's Educational Series.

France, David. 2000. The HIV disbelievers. *Newsweek*, August 19.

French, Linda. 2005. Fathers can promote breastfeeding. *American Family Physician* 71 (February 1):563–4.

French-American Foundation. 2005. Child care (1988–1993). http://www.frenchamerican.org/./prog_education/childcare.html.

Garelli, Juan Carlos. 2004. A brief sketch of John Bowlby's biography. Buenos Aires Attachment Center. April 2. http://attachment.edu.ar/bio.html.

Gettings, John, and David Johnson. 2005. Wonder women: Profiles of leading female CEOs and business executives. Infoplease.com. http://www.infoplease.com/spot/womenceo1.html.

Gilman, Charlotte Perkins. 1983. From the home. In *Visions of women.* Ed. Linda Bell. Clifton, NJ: Humana Press.

Goodwin, Doris Kearns. 1995. *No ordinary time: Franklin and Eleanor Roosevelt: The home front in World War II.* New York: Touchstone.

Graham, Janis. 1995. Mother's milk: What's it in for baby? *Fit Pregnancy*, Summer:102.

Greenberg, Susan. 1999. Nursing trouble. *Newsweek*, Spring/summer.

Greene, Melissa Faye. 2000. The orphan ranger. *New Yorker*, June 17.

Gurian, Anita. 2004. 'Black-box' warnings on antidepressant medication—The latest updates. NYU Child Center Study Center. October 18. http://www.aboutourkids.org/aboutour/articles/black_box_update.html.

Harrison, Lynda Law. 2001. The use of comfort touching and massage to reduce stress in preterm infants in the neonatal intensive care unit. *Newborn and Infant Nursing Reviews* 1 (4):235–241.

Hartmann, Katherine, M. Viswanathan, R. Palmieri, G. Gartlehner, J. Thorp, and K. Lohr. 2005. Outcomes of routine episiotomy: A systematic review. *Journal of American Medical Association* 293:2141–2148.

Health Canada Food Program. 2002. Health professional advisory: Enterobacter sakazakii infection and powdered infant formulas. July 10. http://www.hc-sc.gc.ca/food-aliment/mh-dm/mhe-dme/e_enterobacter_sakazakii.html.

Hewlitt, Sylvia Ann. 2002. *Creating a life: Professional women and the quest for children*. New York: Miramax Books.

Hochschild, Arlie Russell. 1997. *The time bind: When work becomes home and home becomes work*. New York: Metropolitan Books.

Houppert, Karen. 2000. Where do moms fit in? *Parenting*, June/July.

Ikeda, Daisaku, K. Saito, T. Endo, and H. Suda. 2000. Vol. 1 of *The wisdom of the Lotus Sutra*. Vol. I. Santa Monica, CA: World Tribune Press.

Jacobs, Arlene. 1997. Breastmilk: The white blood. *The Compleat Mother*, 46 (Summer):34.

Johnson, Steven. 2003. Love. *Discover* 24(May):70–76.

Karlson, Elizabeth W., Lisa A. Mandl, Susan E. Hankinson, and Francine Grodstein. 2004. Do breast-feeding and other reproductive factors influence future risk of rheumatoid arthritis?: Results from the nurses' health study. *Arthritis and Rheumatism* 50 (11):3458–3467.

Klaus, Marshall H., J. H. Kennell, and P.H. Klaus. 1995. *Bonding: Building the foundations of secure attachment and independence*. Reading, MA: Addison-Wesley.

Kropotkin, Petr. 1976. *Mutual aid*. Boston: Porter Sargent.

Lasch, Christopher. 1977. *Haven in a heartless world: The family besieged*. New York: W.W. Norton.

———. 1997. *Women and the common life: Love, marriage, and feminism*. Ed. Elisabeth Lasch-Quinn. New York: W.W. Norton.

Lawrence, Ruth. 1999. *Breastfeeding: A guide for the medical profession.* 5th ed. St. Louis: Mosby.

Leopold, Kathryn, and Lauren Zoschnick. 2005. Postpartum depression. OBGYN.net. http://www.obgyn.net/femalepatient/default.asp?page=leopold.

Li, R., Z. Zhao, A. Mokdad, L. Barker, and L. Grummer-Strawn. 2003. Prevalence of breastfeeding in the United States: The 2001 national immunization survey. *Pediatrics* 111 (May):1198–201.

Lieberman, Ellice, K. Davidson, A. Lee-Parritz, and E. Shearer. 2005. Changes in fetal position during labor and their association with epidural analgesia. *Obstetrics and Gynecology* 105 (May):974–982.

Marasco, Lisa, C. Marmet, and E. Shell. 2000. Polycystic ovary syndrome: A connection to insufficient milk supply? *Journal of Human Lactation* 16 (2):143–148.

McCutcheon, Susan. 1996. *Natural childbirth the Bradley way.* Revised edition. New York: Plume.

Mokros, Molly. 2002. Women who want domesticity. *Moxie Magazine.* http://www.moxiemag.com/moxie/articles/perspectives/womenwhowant.html.

Montagu, Ashley. 1959. *Human heredity.* Cleveland: The World Publishing Company.

———. 1961. The origin and significance of neonatal and infant immaturity in man. *Journal of the American Medical Association* 178 (1):126–127.

———. 1965. *Life before birth.* New York: Signet books.

———. 1967. *The American way of life.* New York: G.P. Putnam's Sons.

———. 1970. A scientist looks at LOVE. *Phi Delta Kappan* May: 466–467.

———. 1971. What is a child? *National Elementary Principal* 51 (1): 8–16.

———. 1979. Breastfeeding and its relation to morphological, behavioral, and psychocultural development. *Breastfeeding and food policy in a hungry world.* Ed. Dana Raphael. New York: Academic Press.

———. 1986. *Touching: The human significance of the skin.* 3rd ed. New York: Harper and Row.

———. 1996a. *Ashley Montagu's words of wisdom.* Eds. Tsuyoshi Amemiya and Tsutomu Tanaka. Tokyo: Kinko.

———. 1996b. *The elephant man: A study in human dignity.* 3rd ed. Lafayette, LA: Acadian House.

———. 1999. *The natural superiority of women.* 5th ed. Walnut Creek, CA: Altamira Press.

Montagu, Ashley, and Floyd Matson. 1983. *The dehumanization of man.* New York: McGraw-Hill.

Mother Jones. 1998. Editor's Note: Fire fighting. July/August. http://www.motherjones.com/commentary/ednote/1998/07/klein.html.

Murray, B. 2000. Food for thought: Glucose is good for learning and memory. *Monitor on Psychology* 31 (3).

Newman, Jack and Teresa Pittman. 2000. *The ultimate breastfeeding book of answers.* Roseville, CA: Prima Publishing.

Nightingale, Demetra Smith, and Michael Fix. 2004. Economic and labor market trends. The Future of Children. *Children of Immigrant Families* 14 (Summer):49–59. http://www.futureofchildren.org/information2827/information_show.htm?doc_id=241537.

O'Brien, Regina. 2005. Dream job: Stay-at-home mom. Salary.com. May 14. http://www.salary.com/careers/layoutscripts/crel_display.asp?tab-cre&cat=Cat10&ser=Ser253&part=Par358.

O'Connell, Martin. 2001. Labor force participation for mothers with infants declines for first time, Census Bureau reports. United States Department of

Commerce News. October 18. http://www.census.gov/Press-Release/www/2001/cb01-170.html.

Odent, Michael. 1994. Preventing violence or developing the capacity to love: Which perspective? Which investment? Birth and the Origins of Violence. *Primal Health Research* 2 (Winter). http://www.birthpsychology.com/violence/odent1.html.

Offit, Paul A., Bonnie Fass-Offit, and Louis M. Bell. 1999. *Breaking the antibiotic habit.* New York: John Wiley & Sons.

Pacifiers, Bottles Affect Occlusion in Primary Teeth. 2005. *Journal of American Dental Association* 136 (January):36–7.

Pearson, Allison. 2003. Interview by Bookreporter.com. Author talk. May. http://aolsvc.bookreporter.aol.com/authors/talk-pearson-allison.asp#bio.

Peer, Shanny, Olga Baudelot, and Michelle Neuman. 2004. The French System. Economic Opportunity Institute Blueprint. January. http://www.econop.org/ELC/Proposals/EcolesMaternelles.pdf.

Prescott, James W. 1975. Body pleasure and the origins of violence. *The Bulletin of The Atomic Scientists.* November:10–20. http://www.violence.de/prescott/bulletin/article.html.

Reichl, Ruth. 1998. *Tender at the bone: Growing up at the table.* New York: Broadway Books.

———. 2002. *Comfort me with apples: More adventures at the table.* New York: Random House

Robb, Amanda. 2005. Couples: Happily ever after. *Newsweek*, April 25.

Robertson, Brian. 2003. *Day care deception: What the child care establishment isn't telling us.* San Francisco: Encounter Books.

Roiphe, Anne. 1996. *Fruitful: A real mother in the modern world.* New York: Houghton Mifflin.

Rosack, Jim. 2004. Congress hammers FDA over handling of SSRIs. *Psychiatric News* 39 (October 15):1. http://www.antidepressantsfacts.com/2004-10-15-Congress-hammers-FDA-SSRIs.htm.

Ross, Brian, and Jill Rackmill. 2004. Breast-feeding ads stalled, 'watered down.' *ABC News.com.* June 4. http://abcnews.go.com/2020/story?id=124271&page=1.

Ross, Lillian. 1997. Postpartum dept.: A different kind of mommy track in Central Park. *New Yorker,* July 21.

Rubenstein, Carin. 1998. *The sacrificial mother: Escaping the trap of self-denial.* New York: Hyperion Books.

Sarwar and Botting. 1999. Liquid concentrates are lower in bioavailable Tryptophan than powdered infant formulas, and tryptophan supplementation of formulas increases brain tryptophan and serotonin in rats. *Journal of Nutrition* 129:1692–1697.

Senior Journal.com. 2005. Larger number of grandparents taking care of their grandchildren. February 3. http://www.seniorjournal.com/NEWS/Grandparents/03-22-01GrndPrntCare.htm.

Shostak, M. 1981. *Nisa: The life and words of a !Kung woman.* New York: Random House.

Similac Welcome Addition.com. 2005. Similac Advance formula with iron. http://www.welcomeaddition.com/display.cfm?id=139&sub=176.

Sleek, Scott. 1998. Blame your peers, not your parents, author says. *APA Monitor* 29 (October). http://www.snc.edu/psych/korshavn/peer01.htm.

Small, Meredith F. 1998. *Our babies, ourselves.* New York: Anchor Books.

Stehlin, Dori. 1990. Lactation suppression: Safer without drugs. *FDA Consumer* April. http://www.fda.gov/bbs/topics/CONSUMER/CON00069.html.

Stettler, Nicolas, Virginia A. Stallings, Andrea B. Troxel, Jing Zhao, Rita Schinnar, Steven E. Nelson, Ekhard E. Ziegler, and Brian L. Strom. 2005. Weight gain in the first week of life and overweight in adulthood. *Circulation* 111:1897–1903.

Storr, Anthony. 1988. *Solitude*. New York: Random House.

Taddio, Anna, Joel Katz, A Lane Ilersich, and Gideon Koren. 1997. Effect of neonatal circumcision on pain response during subsequent routine vaccination. *Lancet* 349 (March 1):599–603.

The Tocqueville Connection. 2000. More staff, police, sanctions to combat violence in French schools. January 27. http://www.adetocqueville.com/cgi-binloc/searchTTC.cgi?displayZop+3315.

UNICEF. 2005. Infant and young child feeding and care: Protecting, promoting, and supporting breastfeeding.
http://www.unicef.org/nutrition/index_breastfeeding.html.

U.S. Department of Labor. 2005. *Childcare workers*. Bureau of Labor Statistics. http://www.bls.gov/oco/ocos170.htm.

Viggiano, D., D. Fasano, G. Monaco, and L. Strohmenger. 2004. Breast feeding, bottle feeding, and non-nutritive sucking; effects on occlusion in deciduous dentition. *Archives of Disease in Childhood* 89 (January):1121–1123.

Walker, Marsha. 2003. Commentary on formulas supplemented with DHA and ARA. Kellymom.com. January 7.
http://www.kellymom.com/nutrition/milk/DHA-formula-comments.html.

Watson, DL, RK Bhatia, GS Norman, BA Brindley, and RJ Sokol. 1989. Bromocriptine mesylate for lactation suppression: a risk for postpartum hypertension? *Obstetrics and Gynecology* 74: 573–576.

Wharton, Edith. 2001. *The custom of the country*. New York: The Modern Library.

Woolf, Virginia. 1927. *To the lighthouse*. San Diego: Harcourt.

World Health Organization (WHO). 1994. *Breastfeeding: Training health workers*. Division of Child Health and Development. August. www.who.int.

———. 2004. *Feeding the non-breastfed child 6–24 months of age*. Child and Adolescent Health and Development. http://www.who.int/child-adolescent-health/NUTRITION/global_strategy.htm.

———. 2005. *Enterobacter sakazakii and other microorganisms in powdered infant formula: meeting report, MRA Series 6.* Microbiological Risk Assessment Series, No. 6. ISBN: 92 4 156262 5. http://www.who.int/foodsafety/publications/micro/mra6/en/

Wrong Diagnosis.com. 2003. Prevalence and incidence of food poisoning. May 27. http://www.wrongdiagnosis.com/f/food_poisoning/prevalence.htm.

Yalom, Marilyn. 1997. *A history of the breast.* New York: Ballantine Books.

Zoellner, Tom. 2001. A modern man's guide to day care. *Modern Man,* April 19. http://www.modernman.com/cgi-bin/udt/im.display.printable?client.id=modernman&story.id=72.

Index

978-0-595-33546-6
0-595-33546-2

Printed in the United Kingdom
by Lightning Source UK Ltd.
108121UKS00002B/124

9 780595 335466